2005
Men'sHealth.
TOTAL
FITNESS
GUIDE

RODALE

© 2005 by Rodale Inc.

All rights reserved. No part of this publication may be reproduced or transmitted in any form or by any means, electronic or mechanical, including photocopying, recording, or any other information storage and retrieval system, without the written permission of the publisher.

Men's Health is a registered trademark of Rodale Inc.

Printed in the United States of America
Rodale Inc. makes every effort to use acid-free ∞, recycled paper ♻.

ISBN-13 978–1–59486–085–0
ISBN-10 1–59486–085–8

2 4 6 8 10 9 7 5 3 1 hardcover

Visit us on the Web at www.menshealthbooks.com, or call us toll-free at (800) 848-4735.

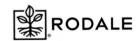

2005 Men's Health
TOTAL FITNESS
GUIDE

EDITOR-IN-CHIEF, *MEN'S HEALTH* MAGAZINE
David Zinczenko

EXECUTIVE EDITOR
Jeremy Katz

EDITOR
Deanna Portz

EXERCISE ADVISOR
Michael Mejia, C.S.C.S.

CONTRIBUTING WRITERS
Mark Anders; Steve Calechman; Adam Campbell; Mary Christ; Alwyn Cosgrove, C.S.C.S.; Jeff Csatari; Ed Eyestone; Brian Good; Carter Hays, C.S.C.S.; Ian King, C.S.C.S.; Joe Kita; Len Kravitz, Ph.D.; Chris Lawson; Michael Mejia, C.S.C.S.; Peter Moore; Myatt Murphy; Scott Quill; Phillip Rhodes; Lou Schuler; Allison Winn Scotch; Ian Smith, M.D.; Ted Spiker; Bill Stieg; Alison Wellner; John R. White, Jr., P.A.-C., Pharm.D.; Mike Zimmerman

INTERIOR DESIGNER
Sandy Freeman

COVER DESIGNER
Christopher Rhoads

PHOTO EDITOR
Darleen Malkames

ASSOCIATE PHOTO EDITOR
Robin Hepler

COPY EDITOR
David Caruso

PROJECT EDITOR
Marilyn Hauptly

LAYOUT DESIGNER
Keith Biery

PRODUCT SPECIALIST
Brenda Miller

SENIOR MANAGING EDITOR
Chris Krogermeier

CONTENT ASSEMBLY MANAGER
Robert V. Anderson, Jr.

ASSOCIATE CONTENT ASSEMBLY MANAGER
Patricia Brown

VICE PRESIDENT, ART DIRECTOR
Andy Carpenter

MANAGING ART DIRECTOR
Darlene Schneck

VICE PRESIDENT, PUBLISHER, DIRECT RESPONSE BOOKS
Gregg Michaelson

SENIOR DIRECTOR, DIRECT RESPONSE MARKETING
Janine Slaughter

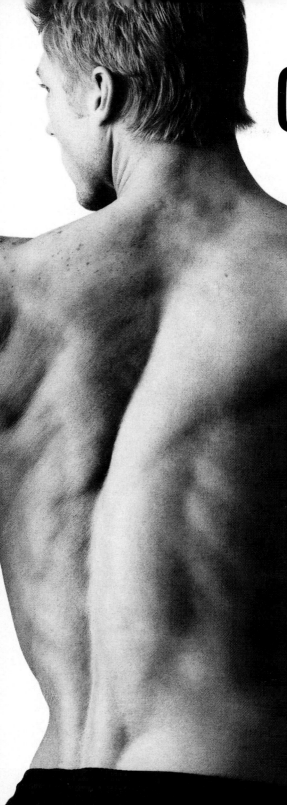

Contents

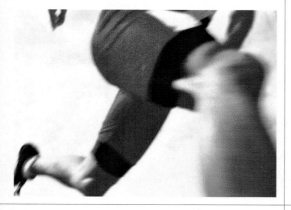

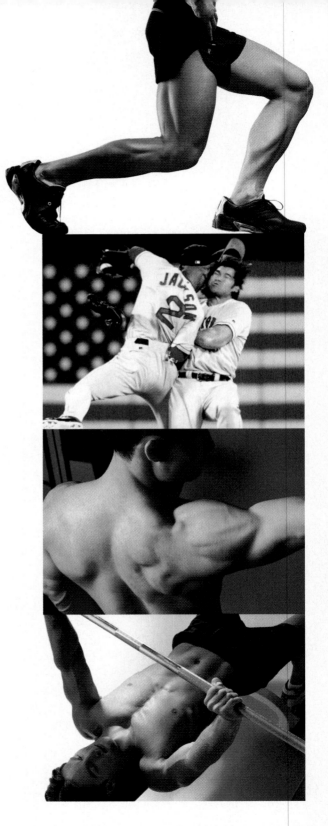

Introduction

Time to Get in Shape

Building your best body takes more than just time. In fact, it shouldn't cost you any time at all. (More on this later.) You need three things to exercise:

- The means
- The energy
- The motivation

Trainers harp on this last point. At my desk at *Men's Health* magazine, I receive a remarkable amount of e-mails and phone calls from trainers—and exercise scientists—who want to let me in on their secret to building a better body: Try harder.

Eureka! (How many advanced degrees did they earn before they realized that?)

Trying harder means different things to different trainers: lift more weight, lift more often, lift weight quickly but lower it slowly, and so on.

But none of this means anything if you don't get to the gym in the first place. Millions of guys are out of shape because they don't go to the gym; and they don't go to the gym because they're out of shape.

You can beat this catch-22, but you have to make the first move. As soon as you notice a change in the way you feel or look, you gain momentum. And the cool thing is, momentum increases fast.

Back to the matter of time. Efficiency experts know we're more productive at work if we take short breaks throughout the day rather than work continuously without rest. The same goes for working out. Pushing yourself too hard, too long is counterproductive. That's why every piece of advice in this book is tailored for guys who don't have an hour every day to work out or to prepare a healthy meal. With these workout strategies, you will make the most of your muscle in the least amount of time. You'll get straightforward nutrition advice to slim down or muscle up. In short, you'll find that getting in your best shape gives you more energy, more motivation, more ambition. Because of this, working out doesn't cost you time, it helps you gain it. As for the means, you don't need a fitness complex in your basement. A gym membership or a few useful tools, such as a set of adjustable dumbbells and a weight bench, makes exercise convenient and easy to stick to.

And don't sweat it whether you're new to training or an ironed vet. The advice here can help any guy.

Now get started, and enjoy your newfound free time—looking and feeling your best.

—SCOTT QUILL

FUEL UP, SLIM DOWN

George Sheehan—the famed cardiologist, runner, and philosopher—once wrote, "Everyone is an athlete. The only difference is that some of us are in training and some of us are not."

Whether or not *you're* in training, you need to eat like you are. Pro athletes use their spring training as a chance to trim excess pounds and fine-tune their muscle-building diets—two things every guy trying to get in shape should do.

This section gives you the tools—workouts and meal plans—to help you get in your best game shape. And like an athlete, you'll be eating plenty of food, with five or six meals a day. No starvation. Ever.

Sound like a weight-loss plan you can sink your teeth into? Yeah, we thought so. Now grab a fork, and start chowing down.

BY LOU SCHULER

You're Fueling Yourself

If you're still following the old rules of weight loss, it's no wonder you haven't had much success. Here's a new way that works

If there's a god of weight loss, he's probably laughing.

For the past 40 years, virtually every weight-loss model has been based on the same principles, and virtually all of them have been wrong. The experts intoned, "Eat less, exercise more." They said that weight loss is all about "calories in, calories out." They informed us that a pound of fat contained roughly 3,500 calories, so if you simply deleted 500 calories from your daily meals or increased your daily exercise by 500 calories, or some combination thereof, you'd lose a pound of fat a week. And if you wanted to lose 2 pounds a week, you just had to double your savings to 1,000 calories a day.

Which is exactly how an anorexic would approach the problem: Starve and strain until you get that perfect, fat-free body, regardless of the muscle you lose or the damage you inflict on your metabolism. And if Lara Flynn Boyle has the body you want, go right ahead and try it.

For the benefit of the rest of you, I want to make two arguments, supported by the latest nutrition and exercise science. That science points toward a new, improved approach to weight loss. First, I want to show that *when* you eat has a profound effect on how your body deals with the calories you feed it. And I want to present a more sophisticated approach to exercise. This approach not only preserves your body's metabolism, the key to weight control, but also makes more productive use of your precious time and energy.

Grab a bite to eat, then chew on this.

Energy Balance Is the Key to Weight Control

If you want to understand energy balance in an instant, think of your body as a car that operates 24 hours a day, says Dan Benardot, Ph.D., R.D., a nutrition researcher at Georgia State University in Atlanta. You would never expect your car to get you from one place to the next without systematic re-fueling, just as you know there's no point in putting more gas in the tank than it's designed to hold. But that's how many of us operate our bodies.

We try to run on empty for hours, then dump in more fuel than we can handle. Benardot's research shows how self-destructive this strategy is.

Let's say you really want to lose fat, and you decide to jog first thing in the morning, on an empty stomach. "The easiest way to get energy is to break down muscle mass," Benardot says. Your body can convert specific amino acids—the building blocks of muscle—to glucose, the sugar that powers human activity. "Someone running before eating may actually be breaking down the very tissue he's trying to improve. Sounds counterproductive to me."

Call it the "muscle loss" diet.

The second way is probably more typical of most of us. You can call this one the "fat gain" diet. You wait a long time between meals, and then, when you're ravenously hungry, you wipe out an entire buffet line. This guarantees that you'll get a larger surge of the hormone insulin than you ordinarily would. That means more fat storage.

And you can probably combine the "muscle loss" and "fat gain" strategies and

Perfect Meal Timing

When you exercise affects what you should eat and when you should eat it. Here's a great meal-planning system, courtesy of Mark Verstegen, a trainer of elite athletes (including Nomar Garciaparra) and author of *Core Performance* (Rodale Inc., January 2004).

	IF YOU WORK OUT IN THE MORNING	IF YOU WORK OUT AT LUNCH	IF YOU WORK OUT RIGHT AFTER WORK
MEAL 1	Preworkout snack: 1/2 whey-protein shake (or) banana and hard-boiled egg (or) cereal w/skim milk	Breakfast: scrambled eggs w/whole-grain toast (or) oatmeal w/crushed flaxseeds and yogurt	Breakfast: scrambled eggs w/whole-grain toast (or) whole-grain cereal w/blueberries and skim milk
MEAL 2	Breakfast (immediately following workout): egg-white omelette w/vegetables, oatmeal, and orange juice	Midmorning/preworkout snack (no more than 1 hour before workout): whey-protein shake w/fruit	Midmorning snack: whey-protein shake w/peanut butter (or) yogurt and cashews
MEAL 3	Midmorning snack: yogurt and fruit (or) whey-protein shake and fruit	Lunch (immediately following workout): chicken-breast sandwich on Kaiser roll and fruit	Lunch: chicken breast, steamed vegetables, and roll
MEAL 4	Lunch: salad w/grilled chicken and olive oil–based dressing (or) tuna or lunchmeat sandwich on whole-grain bread	Midafternoon snack: peanut butter or cashews and an apple (or) meal-replacement bar such as Balance Bar (or) jerky	Midafternoon snack: peanut butter or cashews and an apple (or) meal-replacement bar such as Balance Bar (or) jerky
MEAL 5	Midafternoon snack: peanut butter or cashews and an apple (or) meal-replacement bar such as Balance Bar (or) jerky	Dinner: hamburger made w/ground sirloin (90% lean) or turkey on whole-grain bun and cucumber-tomato salad drizzled w/olive oil	Preworkout snack: 1/2 whey-protein shake
MEAL 6	Dinner: grilled salmon, chicken breast, or sirloin steak and green salad w/olive oil–based dressing		Dinner: grilled salmon, chicken breast, or sirloin steak, green salad w/olive oil–based dressing, and wild rice

turn your body into a perfect muscle-burning, fat-storing machine. Hard exercise slows down appetite in the short term, but as you get used to it, your appetite matches your exertion level. So if you go out and run 10 miles on an empty stomach, then eat enough to fuel a 15-mile run, the net effect is that you've lost muscle on the run and gained fat from the post-run meal.

Energy balance, the focus of Benardot's research, is the answer to both of these dilemmas. The athletes in his studies get the best results when they stay within 300 to 500 calories of perfect energy balance throughout the day. This means . . .

1. Eat as soon as you wake up in the morning.

2. Make sure you eat something before you exercise, no matter what time of day it is. (See "Perfect Meal Timing," on opposite page, for tips on what to eat before exercise.) Not only does the food prevent your muscle tissue from becoming cardio chow, but it increases the number of calories you burn during and after exercise. A 1992 study at Arnot-Ogden Medical Center in Elmira, New York, shows that exercise following a meal enhances metabolism.

3. Eat soon after exercising, when your body has depleted its energy stores. Act fast, or you'll start burning muscle for energy.

4. Eat a total of five or six small meals a day. One of Benardot's studies showed that athletes who added three daily snacks to their three squares lost fat and gained muscle, on top of improving in all the other things that are important to athletes, such as

power and endurance. Of course, you can't simply add a few hundred calories to your diet and lose weight, but you can redistribute your daily calories so you're eating more often but consuming less at individual meals.

However you do it, it's clear to Benardot that the worst strategy is cutting out tons of calories indiscriminately in hopes of sudden, dramatic weight loss. "If you're more subtle and try to lose a pound a week or a pound in 2 weeks, not only can you do it, but you'll be less likely to regain the weight," he says.

10 Pounds of Fat

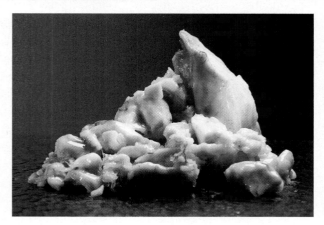

According to a Gallup poll, the average man believes he's overweight by the equivalent of this pile of lard. He's right, and it's likely gathering around his gut. Sure, he can easily hide it under a sweater, but abdominal fat is the worst kind, surreptitiously releasing fatty acids and other toxic substances that increase your risk of disease. Make that 39 diseases. Maybe you ought to nip this in the bud, huh?

Energy Flux Drives Your Metabolism

You probably know that your resting metabolism—the number of calories you burn in the 23 hours a day when you aren't exercising—slows as you get older. That's the reason most of us gain weight as we age. However, a 2001 University of Colorado study found that older men who exercise and eat as much as younger men have similar metabolic rates.

This doesn't mean you have to work out the way you did a decade ago, or that you can drop your Healthy Choice dinners in favor of the Big Macs of your youth. It just

---

Fat? Just Say "Moo"

The obesity epidemic could be put out to pasture if humans simply ate and drank more dairy products. The secret: calcium.

Researchers at Harvard Medical School and elsewhere showed that those who ate three servings of dairy a day, which in conjunction with other foods provides about 1,200 milligrams (mg) of calcium, were 60 percent less likely to be overweight. Go bovine and you'll also have less risk of developing insulin resistance, a precursor to diabetes and heart disease.

Dairy calcium, like strength

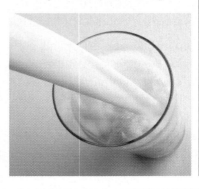

training, helps you burn more calories through inefficiency. You burn more calories digesting calcium-rich foods than you would if you ate something with equal calories but no calcium. The effect is huge. "You're shifting energy away from your fat tissue and toward skeletal muscle for beneficial purposes," says Michael Zemel, Ph.D., director of the Nutrition Institute at the University of Tennessee and author of *The Calcium Key*.

"If you take away only 500 calories a day, the addition of the dairy can approximately double the rate of weight loss," he says. In practical terms, this means losing 2 pounds of fat a week for the price of 1. (Calcium supplements can also help, but they have less than half the power of dairy, Zemel says.)

Try to take in 1,200 mg calcium a day. Some dairy foods that will help:

1 oz grated Parmesan cheese (314 mg)

1 cup large-curd cottage cheese (126 mg)

6-oz Dannon Fruit on the Bottom yogurt (200 mg)

8 oz low-fat milk (264 mg)

1 oz Swiss cheese (1-inch cube; 224 mg)

1 oz Cheddar cheese (204 mg)

1 oz mozzarella cheese (143 mg)

1 scoop Nitro-Tech whey-protein powder (140 mg)

2 scoops vanilla ice cream* (each scoop is ½ c, which is the size of a tennis ball; 184 mg)

12-oz McDonald's Triple Thick vanilla milkshake (350 mg)

1 Dairy Queen Chocolate Dilly Bar (100 mg)

* The New Zealand Ice Cream Company (www.nzicecream.co.nz) makes a calcium-fortified French vanilla dessert with 260 mg calcium per two scoops.

means that the number of calories coming into your body has an influence on the number of calories going out. Two mechanisms are at work.

The first is what textbooks call the "thermic effect of feeding"—the caloric cost of digesting the food you eat. On average, it accounts for about 10 percent of the total calories you burn each day. But that's just an average. It can dip if you eat less, and it can rise if you eat more, or eat more often, or eat different types of foods.

The second mechanism at work is the effect of exercise and other movement throughout the day. This is the part of the equation most weight-loss experts focus on. But if you combine increased feeding with increased movement, you increase your "energy flux," and this is the key to maintaining a fast, muscle-friendly, fat-starving metabolism.

It's no more complicated than balancing your checkbook, which (in my experience, anyway) is a lot easier to do when you have plenty of money coming in than it is when you're unemployed. Some types of food are better at creating energy flux than others. Protein, for example, takes more calories to digest than either carbohydrates or fat. And studies show that protein from animal sources (steak!) seems to have a bigger bang than soy protein (tofu).

The type of exercise you do also affects energy flux. Strength training, for example, can create enormous increases in your resting metabolic rate that last a day or two after your workout. Aerobic exercise doesn't do

20 Pounds

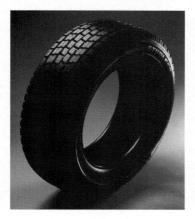

More than 60 percent of American men eat what they want, when they want, according to a Roper survey. No wonder millions of them are an all-conditions radial over their ideal body weight. If that's you, your chances of developing high blood pressure and diabetes are 70 and 250 percent greater, respectively. Now the good news: Losing 10 percent of your body weight is a simple matter of eating smarter and exercising more. Start now and you'll kick the tire in no time.

much, if anything, to boost your metabolic rate, beyond the calories you burn while aerobicizing and for a brief time afterward.

This brings up the obvious question: What is it about strength training that creates a multiday afterburn? The most important factor is muscle repair. An hour of iron therapy causes your muscle tissues to break down at a higher rate than normal. But, thanks to the protein you've eaten after your workout, your muscles are also rebuilding themselves faster than they ordinarily would. So you have energy flux going on within the muscles themselves. A 2003 Finnish study found that protein synthesis (the process that builds bigger muscles) increases by 21 percent 3 hours after a workout, while protein breakdown increases 17 percent. The combination is called "protein turnover," and it uses up a lot of energy.

The type of workout that raises metabolism in studies is usually long and hard, although a recent Ohio University study used a short-but-hard workout and got similar results. The men in the study did circuits of power cleans, bench presses, and squats (a circuit being one exercise right after the other) for 31 minutes. They were still burning more calories than normal 38 hours after the workout.

Inefficient Diet and Exercise Turn Your Body into a Fat-Burning Machine

Efficiency is a good thing when you're talking about running a business. But it

---

Planned Inefficiency: The Workout

No single workout is going to work forever, but this one should keep you busy for the next 2 months. It uses a combination of big-muscle exercises—creating more opportunity for your body to burn calories through the normal muscle-repair process—and inefficient exercises, which burn more calories while you're doing them. It's written for beginners or guys who have let their muscles grow depressingly efficient; more advanced lifters can feel free to substitute the exercises shown in parentheses.

MONDAY, FRIDAY
DO 6 TO 8 REPETITIONS of each exercise in each superset, with little or no rest in between. Rest 60 seconds after completing both exercises. Do each superset two to four times, then move on to the next.

Superset 1
Leg press (barbell squat)
Leg curl (stiff-legged deadlift)

Superset 2
Barbell shoulder press (barbell clean and press)
Lat pulldown (pullup or chinup)

Superset 3
Barbell bench press (barbell wide-grip bench press)
Seated cable row (barbell wide-grip bent-over row)

Superset 4
Situp, with your arms at your sides, across your chest, or behind your head—whichever way allows you to achieve fatigue in 6 to 8 repetitions (weighted situp)

Back extension (weighted back extension)

WEDNESDAY
DO 10 TO 12 REPETITIONS of each exercise in a circuit, with little or no rest in between. Rest 1 to 2 minutes after completing the circuit, then repeat one or two times.

Dumbbell lunge (same, holding weights overhead)
Dumbbell clean and press (same, but press the weights explosively, rising up on your toes)
Dumbbell squat (dumbbell jump squat)
Bench dip (parallel-bar dip)
Reverse pushup (reverse pushup with feet on bench or Swiss ball)
Bicycle crunch (same)

sucks the benefits out of your diet and workout. The more efficient your body is at exercise, the fewer calories it burns. Think of the guy in your health club who does the exact same workout every time you see him, with the exact same weights. He never looks better from one year to the next because his body has become so efficient at doing those moves that it doesn't need to grow bigger muscles or burn more fat in order to finish the workout.

Science has shown us some good strategies for making exercise less efficient:

Strength training. You can make your lifts less efficient in two ways—by increasing the amount of weight you're lifting, or by choosing exercises that are more challenging to your balance and coordination.

Let's say your maximum bench press is 200 pounds. Lifting 200 pounds once is very inefficient; your body throws every muscle fiber into it. But lifting 50 pounds four times is very easy, and thus efficient. The metabolic cost of lifting 200 pounds once is thus greater than the cost of lifting 50 pounds four times. Doing maximum-effort sets of three to six repetitions with, say, 165 to 185 pounds would be a better way to overload your metabolism than doing sets of 10 to 12 reps with lighter weights.

The least efficient lifts are those in which the weight is over your head. This would include standing shoulder presses, as well as exercises such as squats or lunges in which you hold a weight overhead. So instead of doing shoulder presses in a machine or sitting on a bench, stand and crank them out.

30 Pounds

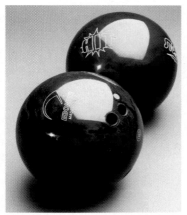

Try carrying a bowling ball around for an hour. Then imagine lugging two of them 24/7, which is exactly what you're asking of your body. No wonder your heart is working overtime and your cholesterol, likely 250 or greater, is in the gutter. If a heart attack strikes today, you have a 16 percent chance of not waking up. You need to begin losing weight now—there is no time to spare. Start with the workout program at the bottom of page 8.

Endurance exercise. No surprises here: If you perform intervals, in which you go hard, then easy, then hard again, you take the efficiency out of your run, swim, or ride. You can call this the "Old Science of Weight Loss," since studies have shown the fat-burning benefits of intervals since the early '90s.

Your diet, too, can be made less efficient, and thus more calorically costly. I showed in the previous section how a higher-protein diet kicks up your metabolism, a sign that your body is burning calories inefficiently. But if that protein comes in the form of high-calcium dairy—milk, yogurt, cheese—you take the inefficiency one giant step further. (See "Fat? Just Say 'Moo'"on page 6.)

50 Pounds

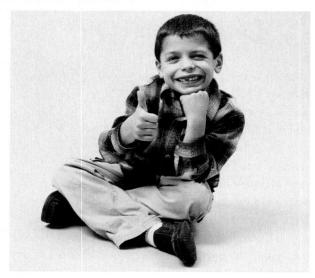

Carry this much extra weight and your chance of dying during your first heart attack is the flip of a coin. Survived the first one? You have a 49 percent chance of having another. Other diseases have your number, too: Your risk of diabetes is up 1,000 percent, and you're 17 percent more likely to suffer a stroke. You're a time bomb, which is too bad for you and the little boy. No, not the one on your gut; the one you'll be leaving fatherless if you don't act today.

Put It All Together Now

That's a lot of science, which I now give you permission to forget. Just remember these five rules that derive from it.

1. Eat five or six times a day, avoiding large gaps between meals and snacks. Don't allow yourself to get ravenously hungry, and don't stuff yourself. If you find you're slipping into a bad mood before a meal, that's a pretty good sign you've waited too long to eat.

2. Eat some protein at every meal and snack, and some calcium-rich dairy at several of them.

3. Always eat something shortly before exercising; you'll burn more calories that way. (See "Perfect Meal Timing" on page 4 for suggestions.) Then eat something soon after. This will speed up the repair process, which also costs your body some caloric capital.

4. Lift weights two to four times a week, focusing on the largest muscle groups. Three total-body workouts a week is ideal for creating a metabolic challenge; that way, you use all your big muscles every time you hit the gym.

5. Try to do something active on two or three of your nonlifting days. If you have the energy, interval workouts are best. But if these additional workouts leave you feeling wiped, it's far better to conserve your energy for three tough strength workouts a week, rather than spread it out over six half-assed exercise sessions.

I wish I could conclude this by telling you that weight loss is fast and easy, rather than slow and strenuous. But the exciting news is that science has found a straighter path to steady, successful weight loss— no starvation or death marches required. Here's wishing you a happy, less efficient new year.

BY ALLISON WINN SCOTCH

What's Sabotaging Your Diet?

Most get-in-shape strategies
are sunk before they can work.
Dive into our simple plan that
identifies—and eliminates—the
culprits keeping you plump

Blame is tricky. When your boss says, "We're not here to assign blame," duck. When we say you're not entirely to blame for your paunch, you're not off the hook. Nobody is the innocent victim of a drive-thru feeding. But there are sneaky factors—your friends, your family, your mind-set—that can sabotage the best weight-loss plan. Your strategy: Identify the saboteurs, then adjust.

The Saboteur: Your wife

We do not suggest blaming her for your belly. This would be (a) wrong and (b) a reasonable defense at her trial. But know this: Researchers at the University of Minnesota found that men and women usually gain 6 to 8 pounds in the first 2 years of marriage. "Once you're married, that need to impress is gone," says Edward Abramson, Ph.D., author of *Marriage Made Me Fat*. "You may go to the gym less often, go out for meals or to parties more frequently, and develop new rituals, such as sitting on the couch with your wife and snacking."

Fix your head: Regain that need to impress. Imagine what that girl at the gym thinks of your gut—or what she'd think if you had abs. (Just don't hit on her.) As for that bowl of popcorn with your wife, Abramson says to ask yourself, "Why am I eating? Boredom? Habit?" Better yet, ask her

to stop bringing those binge foods into the house.

Fix your routine: Establish healthful rituals. Instead of *Access Hollywood* after dinner, take regular walks, or play H-O-R-S-E in the driveway. (P-I-G might work even better.) Exercise suppresses appetite. Cool down with Italian ice (120 calories per cup) instead of ice cream (290 calories per cup).

The Saboteur: Her belly

Dads-to-be gain almost 5 pounds from the end of their partner's pregnancy to the baby's first birthday, Australian researchers report. It's especially common in young, stressed-out fathers, says Lawrence Schwartz, author of *Fat Daddy/Fit Daddy*. And the cycle repeats with each kid.

Fix your head: Be a heroic provider, not a sympathetic eater. Prepare as if fatherhood were a sport—because it will be.

Fix your routine: Read her pregnancy books; they're full of excellent nutritional advice. As for her binge snacking and ice cream jags, adopt a simple policy, says Schwartz: "She can have it, but you shouldn't." Maintain your exercise routine, especially weight lifting. "It's only going to be that much harder to get back into an exercise routine once the baby's here," says Schwartz.

The Saboteur: Your kids

The presence of children in a household sharply increases the likelihood of tempting junk food in the cupboard.

Some of it ends up in adult mouths. Same goes for stray nuggets and fries left over by finicky kids. "I call this 'trolling,'" Schwartz says. "If you're prone to troll, the easiest thing to do is to avoid the Happy Meal altogether."

Fix your head: Grow up. Think: The sugary snack that a child will burn off with an hour of fidgeting will haunt you as a fat deposit. Read the nutrition label on any snack before unwrapping it. Realize the importance of setting a good food-and-exercise example.

Fix your routine: Make junk food a once-a-week thing. Designate Friday as Twinkie day. And instead of standing on the sidelines to watch your son's game, volunteer to coach, ump, or ref. Make fitness a family thing.

The Saboteur: Craig Kilborn

Not getting enough deep, non-REM sleep inhibits production of growth hormone, which might lead to premature middle-age symptoms—abdominal obesity, reduced muscle mass and strength, and diminished exercise capacity. You become Homer Simpson.

Fix your head: "Mentally disengage yourself before you hit the sack," says Jim Karas, author of *The Business Plan for Your Body*. Don't plot a staffing reorg before bed.

Fix your routine: Exercise in the morning or afternoon, says Eric Nofzinger, M.D., director of sleep neuroimaging research at the Western Psychiatric Institute in Pittsburgh. Evening workouts may leave you too stimulated to sleep. Establish a ritual that signals your body that the day is over 30 minutes before bedtime—turn off the computer, read, stretch, or set the TV volume low, says Karas.

The Saboteur: Your shift

Workers gain 7 pounds on average when they switch from a day to a night shift, according to the New York Obesity Research Center. Men working the graveyard shift tend to eat a big evening meal and go to work, says Jim Waterhouse, Ph.D., author of *Keeping in Time with Your Body Clock*. "Then they come home to another 'supper' in the morning."

PEAK performance

Exercise Your Options

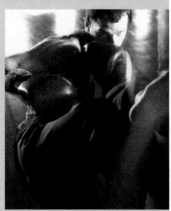

Another reason to switch things up at the gym: According to a new study from the University of California at San Francisco, by the time you reach middle age, your body may actually burn fewer calories doing the same activities that helped keep you lean when you were young. "Both humans and mice gain weight during middle age," says Laurence Tecott, Ph.D., the study author. "We found that the physical activity of mice becomes more energy-efficient at this time—they get more miles to the gallon." A similar process could contribute to obesity in middle-aged men, he says. Tecott suggests it may one day be possible to design drugs to keep the body's calorie-burning powers at their peak.

Fix your head: Adjust your concept of mealtime, says Waterhouse.

Fix your routine: Eat your biggest meal when you get home from your shift, Waterhouse says, then relax or exercise in the morning. Get 8 hours of sleep in the afternoon, then wake up and have breakfast. Kicking off your workday (even if it starts in the evening) with a light meal that's high in protein or fiber is crucial for weight loss.

The Saboteur: Your stress

Stress will spike levels of the hormone cortisol, which tells your body to store fat. "Unfortunately, some people appease their anxiety by reaching for fatty foods," says Elissa Epel, Ph.D., an assistant professor of psychiatry at the University of California at San Francisco. Eating boosts insulin levels; combining that with cortisol leads to greater fat deposits. More stress, bigger belly.

Fix your head: First, identify the type of stress you're under, Karas says. "Is it temporary, like a bar exam, or more permanent, like your job?" Short-term stress will pass. Long-term stress may require a permanent solution, like a new job.

Fix your routine: Make healthy eating effortless, Karas says. Buy snacks that won't send insulin levels soaring: high-fiber energy bars or single-serving bags of almonds or cashews. Fifteen minutes of explosive activity—hitting a speed bag or jumping rope—can alleviate anxieties after work. "It's about getting the tension out," he says.

The Saboteur: Your friends

Buddies can make or break a diet or workout plan, whether it's unconscious scarfing of nachos during the game or the lure of pumping beers instead of iron. Worse, some guys will deliberately try to sabotage your diet, just for sport. Want a cookie?

Fix your head: Admit you need support. "Let people know how to help you, and many will," says Beth Kitchin, an assistant professor of nutritional sciences at the University of Alabama at Birmingham.

Fix your routine: Eat a protein bar before meeting friends, so you'll feel fuller. Drink a glass of water for every glass of beer. A time-tested strategy: Recruit a friend to diet or work out with you. Having someone to answer to is the best enforcement plan.

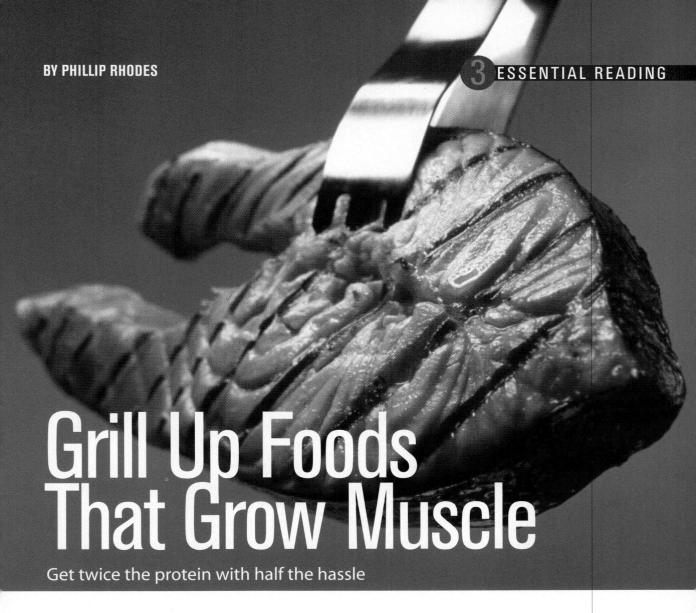

Grill Up Foods That Grow Muscle

Get twice the protein with half the hassle

Your weekend is a great power source. If you play it right, you come out of it recharged and ready for anything. Maybe you'll be a little sore, but that shows you made the most of your days off.

Come spring, even your weekend grilling can serve you well. (Or if you're like us and never cover your grill in the winter, you can benefit right now.) Just buy twice as much of whatever meat or fish you're grilling, and wrap up the extra after you've cooked it. This is power food that will remind you of the wonderful weekend and give you the muscle-repairing protein you need.

We're not talking leftovers here, sputtering back to reheated life in a microwave.

15

Call it "repurposed surplus" brought back in a delicious new setting. Salmon steaks become spicy quesadillas; flank steak morphs into a Thai salad. You're firing up the grill anyway—make the most of your effort.

Salmon Steak

Omega-3-rich salmon steaks hold up well on the grill. Plus, since they're usually sliced to a uniform thickness, they cook evenly. Before you light the fire, coat the rack with cooking spray so the fish won't stick to it.

TODAY: YOSEMITE SALMON

What you'll need:

1 Tbsp smoked paprika

1 tsp black pepper

1 tsp salt

4 salmon steaks, or a full fillet cut into $3^1/_2$-ounce steaks

About 4 tsp honey

How to make it: Mix the spices together in a small bowl. Rub the mixture evenly over the salmon. Grill for 5 minutes per side, drizzling lightly with a squeeze from the honey bear (about 1 tsp per steak) just before they're done. Wrap two steaks and put them in the fridge for tomorrow.

Per serving: 190 calories, 23 grams (g) protein, 7 g carbohydrates, 7 g fat (1 g saturated), less than 1 g fiber, 630 milligrams (mg) sodium

Eat with: Grilled corn on the cob. Brush the ears lightly with olive oil and grill for about 10 minutes, turning frequently. Serve with a lime wedge.

TOMORROW: SALMON QUESADILLAS

What you'll need (per quesadilla):

2 8" whole-wheat tortillas

$^3/_4$ c shredded low-fat Cheddar or Monterey Jack cheese, divided

1 leftover salmon steak, flaked

$^1/_2$ c Mexicorn, drained

$^1/_4$ c chopped green onion

$^1/_2$ tsp red-pepper flakes

How to make it: Heat a cooking spray–coated nonstick skillet over medium heat. When it's hot, place the first tortilla in the skillet. Sprinkle on half of the cheese. Add remaining ingredients. Top with the remaining cheese and the second tortilla. Cook, pressing down occasionally with a spatula, for 6 to 8 minutes, or until the cheese melts and the tortilla starts to become crisp. Flip and cook for about 6 minutes more.

Per serving: 430 calories, 40 g protein, 53 g carbohydrates, 11 g fat (3 g saturated), 6 g fiber, 980 mg sodium

Eat with: Salsa

Flank Steak

Flank steak must be tender. Marinate it in a mixture that contains acidic liquid like citrus juice, vinegar, or wine. Don't overcook it—medium rare, max. Let it stand 5 minutes before you slice it, so the juices have time to settle into the meat. And last, slice it across the grain on a diagonal to further break down the meat's structure.

TODAY: BASIC BALSAMIC FLANK STEAK

What you'll need:

1 whole flank steak (1¹/₂ lb)

Marinade made with ²/₃ c balsamic vinegar; 1 Tbsp black pepper; 2 cloves garlic, crushed

How to make it: Poke the meat with a fork to help the marinade penetrate. Mix the marinade in a large resealable bag, reserving ¹/₄ cup. Drop the steak into the bag and refrigerate it for up to 24 hours. Grill for 6 to 8 minutes per side (until medium rare). Brush with the reserved marinade before serving. Slice diagonally across the grain in thin slices. Reserve half the steak, unsliced, for tomorrow. Once it's cool, wrap it tightly in plastic wrap and refrigerate.

Per serving: 360 calories, 48 g protein, 8 g carbohydrates, 14 g fat (6 g saturated), 0 g fiber, 105 mg sodium

Eat with: Potato wedges. Quarter 2 potatoes lengthwise, coat with cooking spray, then sprinkle lightly with garlic powder and dried or fresh rosemary. Grill, turning occasionally, for 15 to 20 minutes or until tender.

TOMORROW: THAI SALAD

What you'll need:

6 big handfuls mixed greens

¹/₂ red bell pepper and ¹/₄ red onion, both sliced in thin strips

1¹/₂ Tbsp chopped fresh basil

³/₄ lb leftover flank steak, sliced thin on the diagonal

Dressing made with (per salad) 2 Tbsp soy sauce; 2 tsp sesame oil;

2 small cloves garlic, crushed; pinch of red-pepper flakes

1 Tbsp chopped peanuts

How to make it: Mix together the greens, bell pepper, onion, and basil. Add the steak. Blend the dressing, and drizzle over the salad. Top with peanuts. Makes 2 servings.

Per serving: 471 calories, 53 g protein, 13 g carbohydrates, 22 g fat (7 g saturated), 5 g fiber, 676 mg sodium

Eat with: Whole-wheat pita chips. Stack 2 pitas and cut into 8 wedges. Spray wedges lightly with cooking spray, and bake them at 350°F for about 10 minutes or until crisp.

Chicken Breasts

Shorten grilling time by pounding the chicken breasts to an even thickness before cooking. Put each breast between sheets of plastic wrap and, starting at the thickest point, pound the chicken with a tenderizer or the heel of your hand until the thick part is even with the thin part. Go ahead—get some aggression out. The chicken's already dead.

TODAY: BEER-B-Q CHICKEN

What you'll need:

4 boneless, skinless chicken breasts

Marinade made with ¹/₂ can beer, ¹/₂ c low-sugar BBQ sauce (like Jim Beam), 1 tsp cayenne pepper

How to make it: Put the chicken in a resealable plastic bag with the marinade, setting aside ¹/₄ cup, and refrigerate overnight. Grill for about 12 to 15 minutes per side.

Brush with the reserved marinade before serving. Wrap two chicken breasts and refrigerate.

Per serving: 180 calories, 27 g protein, 5 g carbohydrates, 3.5 g fat (1 g saturated), 1 g fiber, 105 mg sodium

Eat with: Summer squash. Slice zucchini and yellow squash. Toss in a small handful of slivered almonds. Steam until tender.

TOMORROW: SPICY CHICKEN STEW
What you'll need:
2 leftover chicken breasts, cubed or torn into thin strips
4 c low-sodium chicken broth
1 can diced, no-salt-added tomatoes, liquid included
1/4 c canned jalapeño peppers
1 small can corn, drained
3 cloves garlic, crushed
2 tsp cumin
1 Tbsp chili powder
1 tsp cocoa powder

How to make it: Put everything into a big pot, stir, bring to a boil, then reduce the heat and simmer for 20 minutes uncovered, stirring occasionally. Makes 2 servings.

Per serving: 490 calories, 47 g protein, 66 g carbohydrates, 10 g fat (2.5 g saturated), 11 g fiber, 1,000 mg sodium

Eat with: Baked tortilla chips and guacamole: Peel and pit 3 avocados and mash along with 1 small onion, chopped; 2 Roma tomatoes, chopped; the juice of 1 lime; and 1 tsp salt.

Tuna Steaks
A restaurant chef barely touches a tuna steak to his grill, then serves it almost raw inside. For these recipes, it's okay to cook the tuna through to medium. Otherwise, the juices might soak right through your tortilla when the tuna reappears as a taco filling tomorrow.

TODAY: MEXCELLENT TUNA
What you'll need:
4 1"-thick tuna steaks
Marinade made with 1 c tequila, juice of 1 lime, 1/2 tsp dried cilantro

How to make it: Put the tuna in a resealable bag with the marinade, setting aside 1/4 cup, and refrigerate for 45 minutes. Grill for 4 to 5 minutes per side. Brush with the reserved marinade before serving. Refrigerate two steaks in plastic wrap for tomorrow.

Per serving: 290 calories, 34 g protein, 1 g carbohydrates, 1.5 g fat (0 g saturated), 0 g fiber, 55 mg sodium

Eat with: Mixed green salad

TOMORROW: TUNA TACOS
What you'll need (per taco):
Half a leftover tuna steak, cubed
Handful of bagged coleslaw mix
1 Tbsp chopped red onion
1 small corn tortilla
1 Tbsp sweet pickle relish, drained
1 Tbsp plain yogurt or mayonnaise

How to make it: Put the tuna into a microwave-safe bowl and zap for 2 minutes,

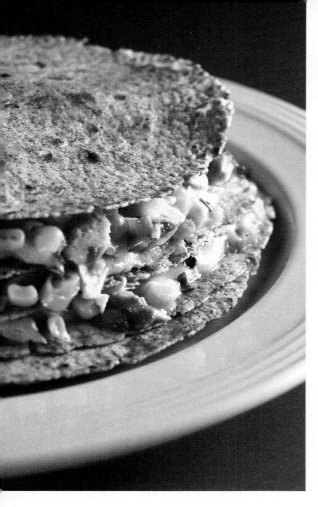

Think of the tender, flavorful meat as veal without the guilt. Bonus: Lamb is a leading source of conjugated linoleic acid (CLA), a fatty acid that's been linked to successful weight loss. In fact, the only meat with more CLA is kangaroo, according to a recent Australian study.

TODAY: BAA BAA AND KEBABS

What you'll need:
1 carton cherry tomatoes
1 carton whole button mushrooms
1 yellow or red bell pepper, chopped
    into large pieces
1 medium red onion, chopped into
    large chunks
1 Tbsp olive oil
$1/2$ tsp cumin
4 lamb chops (about 4 oz each)
Sauce made with 1 c plain low-fat
    yogurt; $1/3$ English cucumber
    (the seedless kind), chopped; 2
    tsp fresh or dried mint, chopped

How to make it: Alternate vegetables on four skewers. Brush them with olive oil and sprinkle lightly with cumin. Grill the kebabs and chops for 5 minutes per side (until the chops are medium rare). Use the sauce for dipping. Reserve two lamb chops, and refrigerate for tomorrow.

Per serving: 355 calories, 27 g protein, 15 g carbohydrates, 21 g fat (8 g saturated), 2 g fiber, 125 mg sodium

Eat with: Couscous (it cooks really quickly)

stirring after 1 minute. Arrange the tuna, slaw, and onion on the tortilla. Top with the relish and yogurt or mayo.

Per serving (two tacos): 337 calories, 39 g protein, 36 g carbohydrates, 3 g fat (0 g saturated), 4 g fiber, 340 mg sodium

Eat with: Low-fat refried beans

Lamb

Lamb deserves a closer look. What beef is to America, lamb (and its grown-up counterpart, mutton) is to Greece, Morocco, New Zealand, and many other parts of the world.

TOMORROW: SA-LAMB BOMBAY

What you'll need:

1 tsp olive oil

1 small onion, chopped

$1/2$ c canned, diced, no-salt-added tomatoes

2 leftover lamb chops, cut into small, bite-size pieces

1 c low-sodium chicken broth

$1/4$ c light coconut milk

1 tsp curry powder

1 tsp dried cilantro

$1/2$ tsp red-pepper flakes

$1^1/2$ Tbsp slivered almonds

How to make it: Heat the oil in a skillet. Add the onion and sauté over medium-low heat until soft (about 5 minutes), stirring occasionally. Add the tomatoes and lamb. Sauté for 2 minutes. Add the chicken broth, coconut milk, spices, and almonds. Stir and bring to a boil. Cook uncovered, stirring occasionally, for 5 to 10 minutes or until the mixture is thick like gravy. Makes 2 servings.

Per serving: 350 calories, 32 g protein, 10 g carbohydrates, 20 g fat (6 g saturated), 3 g fiber, 170 mg sodium

Eat with: Instant brown rice or mashed potatoes

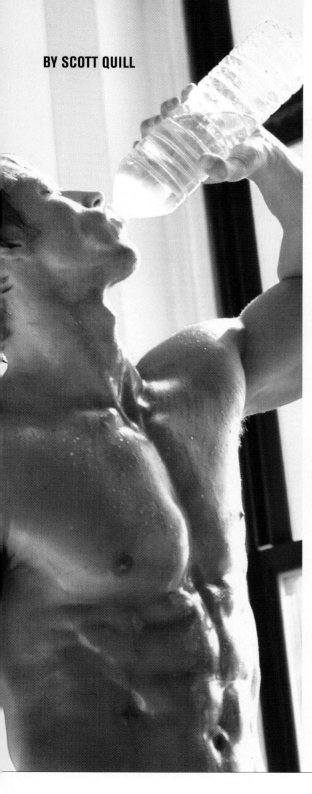

BY SCOTT QUILL

Where There's a Pill, There's a (Better) Way

Before you swallow a weight-loss pill, read our fine print

We know ephedra helps people lose weight. We also know it isn't for everybody, which is why the warning labels told people with high blood pressure, heart disease, and other health problems to stay away. But when Baltimore Orioles pitching prospect Steve Bechler died after using ephedra—even though he ignored warnings that were so specific to his health problems that his picture might as well have appeared on the label—supplement companies knew it was all over. The FDA banned ephedra in December 2003.

But the manufacturers are still selling their products. They've simply reformulated them, promising the same results but with different, "ephedra-free" ingredients. They're telling us we can have our cake and eat it, too, confident that none of those frosting-covered calories will end up hanging over our belts. And even before the FDA ban, we were buying it; in 2002, sales of just one ephedra-free weight-loss supplement totaled $25 million. But what are we really getting for all that green? Science or snake oil? A little of both, it turns out. Here's a sampling of what's inside today's kinder, gentler fat burners.

The Product: Ephedra-Free Hydroxycut

The claim: "Can help increase your body's weight-loss potential . . . and reduce hunger cravings!"

Primary active ingredient: Hydroxycitric acid (amount unknown)

An extract of an Indian fruit called malabar tamarind, hydroxycitric acid (HCA) is touted as a natural appetite suppressant. And that's partly true—it is natural. A study published in the *Journal of the American Medical Association* determined that a 1,500-milligram (mg) daily dose had absolutely no effect on appetite or weight loss. Still, the company cites a study (as yet unpublished) that found

that people who took 2,800 mg HCA every day for 8 weeks lost twice as much weight as those taking a placebo. But experts remain unconvinced. "Having worked with the product, I am skeptical," says James Hill, Ph.D., director of the University of Colorado's center for human nutrition. "It's possible that higher doses have this great effect, but I personally think it's unlikely."

The verdict: Until there's evidence otherwise, drop this acid from your supplement shopping list. Instead, stick with a fruit extract that's a proven hunger squelcher: pectin. Just 5 mg of this gelatinlike substance—the amount in one large apple—has been found to increase satiety and reduce weight, according to research published in the *Journal of the American College of Nutrition*.

The Product: Xenadrine EFX

The claim: "Uses advanced thermogenic technology!"

Primary active ingredient: Thermodyne complex, including green tea extract and caffeine (amounts unknown)

The Chinese have been sipping green tea for thousands of years, so this isn't exactly "advanced" technology. But that aside, a study published in the *American Journal of Clinical Nutrition* did find that when 10 men were given 270 mg EGCG—a chemical found in green tea—and 50 mg caffeine, their metabolisms increased by 4 percent, compared with less than 1 percent when they had the caffeine alone. Over the course of a year, this boost to your fat-burning capacity could translate to an additional weight loss of 12 pounds. The catch? The study only looked at the effects of EGCG and caffeine over the course of a single day. "Green tea extract elevates metabolism over a 24-hour period, but we don't know if this effect continues if you take it every day," says Jose Antonio, Ph.D., C.S.C.S., a nutrition and exercise researcher in Deerfield Beach, Florida.

The verdict: Without knowing the amount of caffeine and green tea in Xenadrine, there's no way to tell if it'll work, be it for a day or a week. A better bet: Shortly before you go to sleep, eat 1 cup of cottage cheese, one of the best sources of a protein called casein. You want casein in your bedtime snack because it reduces catabolism, a process in which your body breaks down muscle tissue instead of fat, while you sleep, says Christopher R. Mohr, M.S., R.D., a nutritionist at the University of Pittsburgh. Retain more muscle and your metabolism will speed up over time, causing you to wake up leaner than when you hit the pillow.

The Product: Trim Spa Completely Ephedra Free

The claim: "Has an ingredient that prolongs the amount of time that food is available for energy, thus keeping it from being stored as fat."

Primary active ingredient: Glucosamine (300 mg)

Yes, the same glucosamine that greases your joints is supposed to shrink your gut.

The theory: Glucosamine, a naturally occurring amino acid derivative, weakens insulin action, which in turn may prevent fat storage. When researchers at the Washington University School of Medicine tested this theory on fat rats, they found that giving the rodents 10 millimoles (mM) of glucosamine increased their insulin resistance by 50 percent. Problem is, 10 mM is enough glucosamine to flood every cell in a rat's body. Now, if you were to try to swallow a proportionate amount of the stuff—well, you couldn't. "The doses used in rodent studies are typically much higher than are used in humans," says Michael Schwartz, M.D., head of the section of clinical nutrition, division of metabolism, endocrinology, and nutrition, at the University of Washington.

The verdict: Save the glucosamine for your bum knee. And if you want to make insulin your ally in your struggle to slim down, choose foods such as low-fat dairy products, fish, lean beef, and nuts instead of munching on white bread and grapes or bananas. These high-protein, low-carb foods help to maximize insulin's appetite-suppressing powers by making you feel fuller longer.

The Product: Prolab Therma Pro Ephedra Free

The claim: "Stimulates metabolic rate and promotes fat loss."

Primary active ingredients: Synephrine (60 mg) and Coleus forskohlii (375 mg)

Synephrine is ephedra's chemical cousin, but it may be a weak sister when it comes to weight loss. In a 6-week study published in *Current Therapeutic Research,* researchers found that people who took synephrine (975 mg), caffeine (528 mg), and St. John's wort (900 mg) daily while also dieting and exercising lost about 3 percent of their body fat, versus no change in those who only dieted and exercised. Not bad, but not necessarily a result of the synephrine, particularly given the megadose of caffeine used. "You can't really say whether it's specifically tied to one of the ingredients or it's a synergistic effect," says Jeff Volek, Ph.D., R.D., an exercise and nutrition researcher at the University of Connecticut. As for Coleus forskohlii, you may burn more calories trying to pronounce the name than you will by taking the stuff; there is virtually no scientific research to support consuming this Indian plant as a way to manage one's weight.

The verdict: Even if synephrine was the force behind the fat loss seen in the study, Prolab's product is about 915 mg shy of the amount the researchers tested. But you can still speed up your metabolism—just eat more fish, especially salmon and tuna. Several studies have shown that the omega-3 fatty acids in fish can help lower the body's blood levels of leptin, a hormone that can keep our metabolisms stuck in first gear.

The Product: Zantrex-3

The claim: "The ultimate appetite suppressant."

Primary active ingredients: Yerba mate, guarana, and damiana (amounts unknown)

This herbal threesome from South America supposedly suppresses your appetite by slowing the digestive process. The evidence: A study published in the *Journal of Human Nutrition and Diet* shows that people who took the combination for 45 days dropped 10 1/2 pounds more than those taking a placebo. Impressive results, until you consider that the researchers neglected one small detail: food, as in the amount and type everyone ate. "You can't measure weight loss without controlling for diet," says Mohr. For all the researchers know, the supplement group was on Atkins and the sugar-pill subjects were carbing it up. But even if you assume that diet wasn't a factor (and you really shouldn't), it's impossible to know whether Zantrex-3 will work, since there's no mention on the bottle of how much yerba mate, guarana, and damiana is in each capsule.

The verdict: Don't bother going below the equator to shorten your own latitudinal lines. Stay put, and time the length of your next meal. "It takes 20 minutes for your brain to recognize that you're full," says Marilyn Tanner, M.S., R.D., a spokeswoman for the American Dietetic Association. If you usually finish in less time, you could be overeating. Can't seem to slow yourself down? Tanner suggests breaking your meals into courses, taking a sip of a low-calorie beverage between bites, and never eating with your fingers—even if it's a finger food. (You can't fit as much on a fork.)

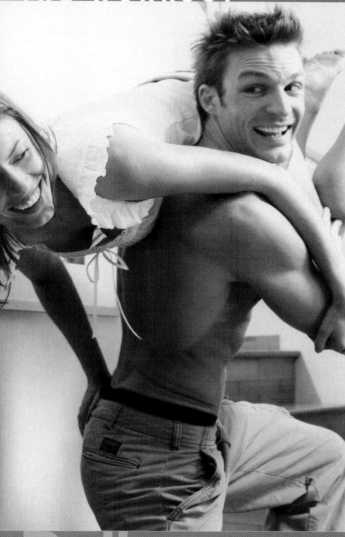

Belly Blaster

Bust your gut with our 4-week fat-melting plan

Even with the low-carb craze, you still haven't given up your roll with dinner? Then you probably have rolls around your middle, too. This fat-burning regimen will help you lose your gut in 4 weeks. So go ahead, have that roll. Just limit it to one.

Instructions

If you belong to a gym, you can do the workouts exactly as shown here. Or, if you work out at home and have limited equipment, you can replace machine exercises with the designated alternate versions.

Do the beginner workout if you have less than a year of strength-training experience, or if you're coming back from a layoff of longer than 4 months. Do the intermediate/advanced program if you've worked out consistently for the past year or longer.

BY MICHAEL MEJIA, C.S.C.S.

Do the beginner workout 2 days a week and the sprint workout on one of the days in between. Perform all the exercises in the beginner workout as a modified circuit, doing one exercise after another with 30 seconds of rest after each move. After you've completed a full circuit, rest for 2 minutes. Then repeat the circuit one or two more times, for a total of two or three sets of each exercise. Do 8 to 15 repetitions in each set.

SPRINT WORKOUT

Warm up for 3 to 5 minutes by running at an easy pace. Then sprint at 95 percent of full effort for 10 to 15 seconds. Rest for 90 seconds, and repeat nine times. Each week, add two more sprints and reduce the rest periods by 10 seconds.

ZERCHER SQUAT

● Hold a barbell in the crook of your elbows, and stand with your feet shoulder-width apart.

● Keeping your torso as upright as possible (lift with your legs, not your back), squat until your thighs are parallel to the floor. Push up through your heels to return to the starting position.

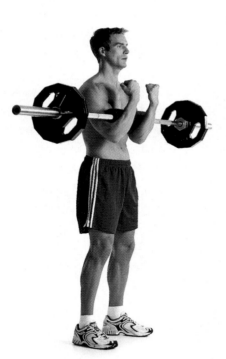
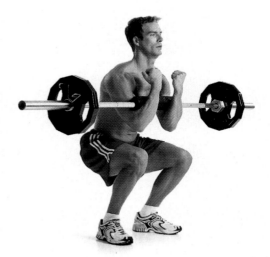

PUSHUP

● Support your body with the balls of your feet and with your hands, positioning the latter slightly wider than shoulder-width apart, palms flat on the floor. Straighten your arms without locking your elbows.

● Lower your torso until your chest is just a fraction of an inch off the floor. Push yourself back to the starting position.

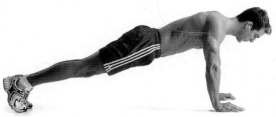

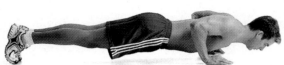

LEG PRESS (Alternate: Step-Up)

● Sit back in a leg-press station with your back against the pad and your feet shoulder-width apart on the foot plate. Adjust the seat so your knees are bent slightly more than 90 degrees.

● Push the weight until your knees are straight but not locked. Pause, then return to the starting position.

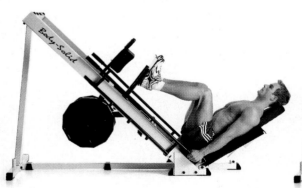

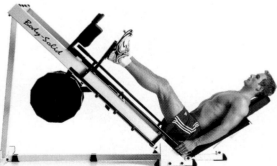

LOW-TO-HIGH CABLE ROW (Alternate: Bent-Over Row)

● Attach a rope handle to a low pulley, and set a pair of 45-pound weight plates on the floor to either side of the pulley. Grab the rope with an overhand grip and sit on the floor about 2½ feet in front of the low pulley, with your arms straight, your feet braced against the weight plates, and your torso erect.

● Start the movement by pinching your shoulder blades together in back, then pull the rope up to just underneath your chin. Keep your elbows up and out. Pause, then slowly return to the starting position.

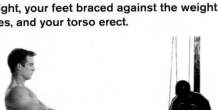
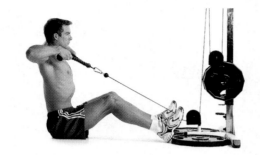

DUMBBELL 45-DEGREE TRAVELING LUNGE

● Stand with your feet hip-width apart, and hold two dumbbells at your sides.

● Lunge-step out at a 45-degree angle—forward and to the side—with your front thigh ending up parallel to the floor and your front knee over your toes. Then step forward with your back foot, so you end up in the starting position a few feet northeast or northwest of where you started. Do the next rep with the other foot, angling toward the other side, like you're doing a drunken wedding march. Keep alternating until you finish your reps—or until you hit a wall.

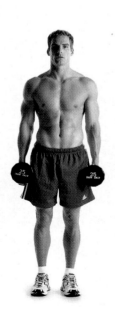
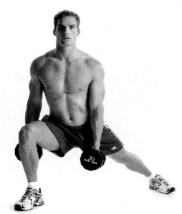

CABLE UPRIGHT ROW (Alternate: Upright Row)

● Attach an EZ-curl bar to the low cable. (A straight bar is okay, although it's not as easy on your wrists.) Stand facing the weight stack, about a foot in front of it. Grab the bar with an overhand, shoulder-width grip, and hold it at arm's length in front of your thighs.

● Pull the bar up until your upper arms are parallel to the floor (no higher). Pause, then slowly lower the bar back to the starting position.

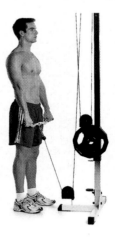

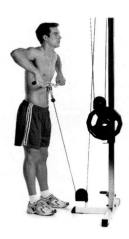

LAT PULLDOWN (Alternate: Pullover)

● Attach a long straight bar to a high cable, and slide a bench underneath it. Sit on the bench, and grab the bar with a false (thumb on the same side as your fingers), overhand, shoulder-width grip. Keep your arms straight and your torso upright or leaning back slightly.

● Pull your shoulder blades together and down, stick your chest out, and pull the bar to your chest. Pause with the bar an inch or two off your chest, then slowly let it rise to the starting position. Keep your chest out.

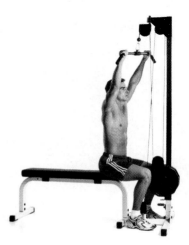

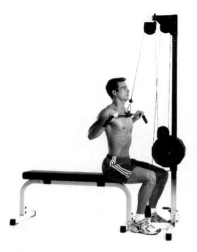

SWISS BALL HIP EXTENSION AND LEG CURL (Alternate: Lying Hip Extension)

● Put your heels and calves on a Swiss ball, and spread your arms on the floor for added stability. Pushing with your gluteals and hamstrings, dig your heels down into the ball, and lift your hips until your body forms a ramp that descends from your knees to your shoulders.

● At the top of the movement, execute a leg curl by using your hamstrings to roll the ball toward your butt. Hold at the point of greatest contraction, straighten your legs, and then lower your body to the starting position.

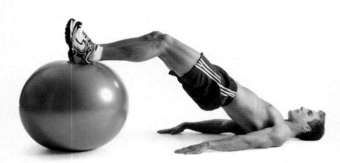
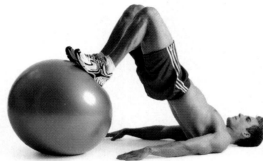

SITUP

● Lie on your back with your knees bent and your feet flat on the floor. Hold your hands behind your ears. (Don't interlock your fingers behind your head.)

● Slowly lift your upper body off the floor by using your abdominals to bring your chest toward your knees. Roll back down, slowly and with control.

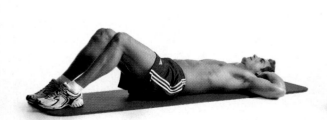
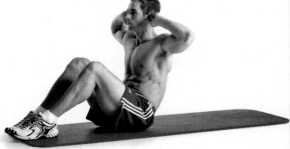

DUMBBELL TWISTING SHOULDER PRESS

● Stand while holding a pair of dumbbells just outside your shoulders at jaw level, palms facing in.

● Press the dumbbells overhead as you twist your torso to your right. Lower the dumbbells back to the starting position as you turn to the center. Turn to the left as you press the weights up again, and lower them as you return to the starting position.

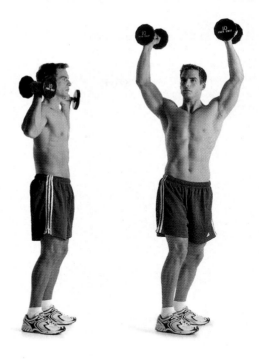

SWISS BALL JACKKNIFE (Alternate: V-Up)

● Get into a pushup position with the tops of your feet and your shins on the ball and your hands on the floor.

● Pull your knees close to your chest, letting the ball roll slightly forward. Keep your arms straight, and squeeze your abs hard at the top.

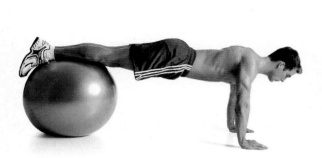

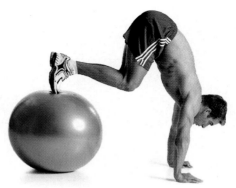

BENCH DIP

● Hold on to the seat of a bench behind you (make sure it's secure and will not move away from you as you dip), with your knees bent and your feet flat on the floor—as if you were seated in an invisible chair in front of the bench.

● Keep your back arched and close to the bench as you slowly lower your body until your upper arms are parallel to the floor. Your torso should remain straight. Pause, then press back up to the starting position.

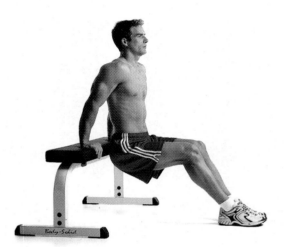
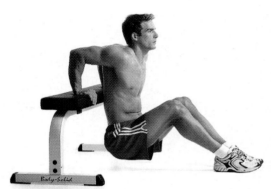

Alternate between workouts A and B each workout, 3 days a week, performing the sprint workout after each session. In workouts A and B, perform each superset—a pair of exercises done as a single set—with no rest between exercises. After completing both exercises, immediately repeat the superset two more times without resting, for a total of three sets of each exercise. Then rest 90 seconds, and begin the exercises in the next superset. For each move, start with a weight you can lift at most 10 times, and do as many reps as you can in each set.

SPRINT WORKOUT

Warm up for 3 to 5 minutes by running at an easy pace. Then sprint at 95 percent of full effort for 10 to 15 seconds. Rest for 90 seconds, and repeat nine times. Each week, add two more sprints and reduce the rest periods by 10 seconds.

WORKOUT A

SUPERSET 1

BARBELL HACK SQUAT

● This move is rough on your knees, so avoid it if you have a history of knee problems. Set a barbell on the floor behind a pair of large weight plates. Stand with your feet about shoulder-width apart and your heels up on the weight plates. Squat down, grab the bar with a shoulder-width, underhand grip, then stand up so the bar rests behind your hamstrings.

● Descend toward the floor with your arms straight and your torso erect. Stop when the tops of your thighs are parallel to the floor and the bar grazes your Achilles tendons. Pause, then return to the starting position.

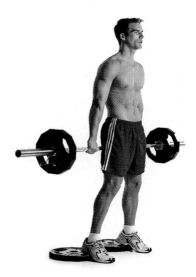

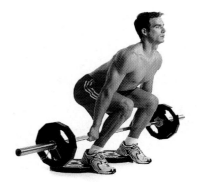

T PUSHUP

● Hold a pair of light dumbbells with a neutral grip (thumb on opposite side of fingers, palms facing in), and get into the down position of a standard pushup, with your hands directly below your shoulders.

● Execute a basic pushup. Then hold the top position, and lift one dumbbell toward the ceiling while rotating your torso in the same direction, so you face to the side. Support and balance yourself with the other arm, so your arms and body form a T, with your arms perpendicular to the floor. Return to the starting position, and repeat with the opposite arm lifting the dumbbell.

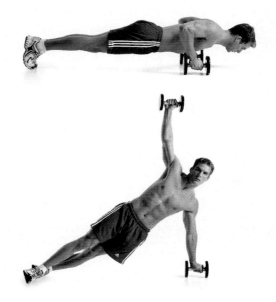

SUPERSET 2

DUMBBELL 45-DEGREE TRAVELING LUNGE

● Stand with your feet hip-width apart, and hold two dumbbells at your sides.

● Lunge-step out at a 45-degree angle—forward and to the side—with your front thigh ending up parallel to the floor and your front knee over your toes. Then step forward with your back foot, so you end up in the starting position a few feet northeast or northwest of where you started. Do the next rep with the other foot, angling toward the other side, like you're doing a drunken wedding march. Keep alternating until you finish your reps—or until you hit a wall.

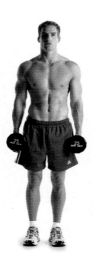

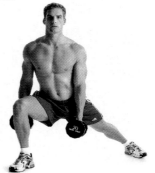

CABLE UPRIGHT ROW (Alternate: Upright Row)

● Attach an EZ-curl bar to the low cable. (A straight bar is okay, although it's not as easy on your wrists.) Stand facing the weight stack, about a foot in front of it. Grab the bar with an overhand, shoulder-width grip, and hold it at arm's length in front of your thighs.

● Pull the bar up until your upper arms are parallel to the floor (no higher). Pause, then slowly lower the bar back to the starting position.

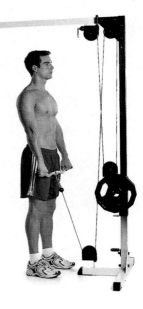 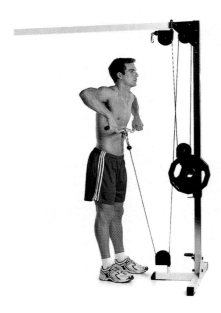

SUPERSET 3

SITUP

● Lie on your back with your knees bent and your feet flat on the floor. Hold your hands behind your ears. (Don't interlock your fingers behind your head.)

● Slowly lift your upper body off the floor by using your abdominals to bring your chest toward your knees. Roll back down, slowly and with control.

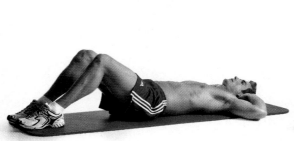 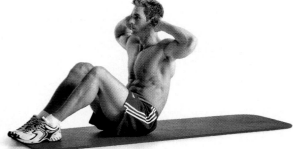

DUMBBELL TWISTING SHOULDER PRESS

● Stand while holding a pair of dumbbells just outside your shoulders at jaw level, palms facing in.

● Press the dumbbells overhead as you twist your torso to your right. Lower the dumbbells back to the starting position as you turn to the center. Turn to the left as you press the weights up again, and lower them as you return to the starting position.

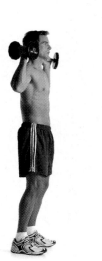
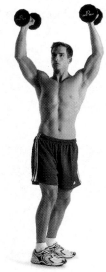

WORKOUT B

SUPERSET 1

WIDE-GRIP PULLUP

● Grab a pullup bar with an overhand grip, placing your hands well outside your shoulders, and hang with your elbows slightly bent.

● Pull your chin above the bar, hold for a second or two, and lower your body with control.

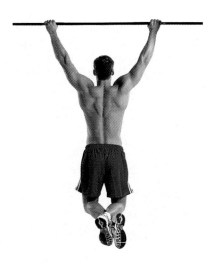
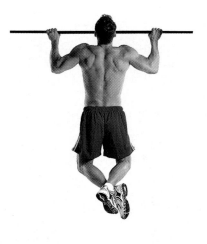

SWISS BALL HIP EXTENSION AND LEG CURL

(Alternate: Lying Hip Extension)

● Put your heels and calves on a Swiss ball, and spread your arms on the floor for added stability. Pushing with your gluteals and hamstrings, dig your heels down into the ball and lift your hips until your body forms a ramp that descends from your knees to your shoulders.

● At the top of the movement, execute a leg curl by using your hamstrings to roll the ball toward your butt. Hold at the point of greatest contraction, straighten your legs, and then lower your body to the starting position.

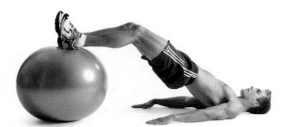 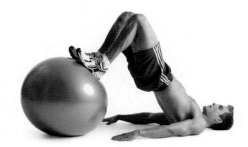

SUPERSET 2

LOW-TO-HIGH CABLE ROW (Alternate: Bent-Over Row)

● Attach a rope handle to a low pulley, and set a pair of 45-pound weight plates on the floor to either side of the pulley. Grab the rope with an overhand grip, and sit on the floor about 2½ feet in front of the low pulley, with your arms straight, your feet braced against the weight plates, and your torso erect.

● Start the movement by pinching your shoulder blades together in back, then pull the rope up to just underneath your chin. Keep your elbows up and out. Pause, then slowly return to the starting position.

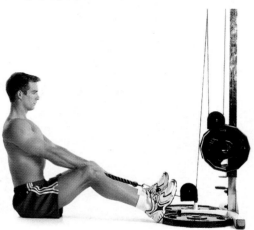 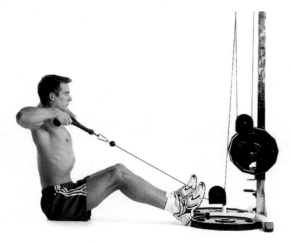

DUMBBELL LUNGE

● Stand with your feet hip-width apart, and hold two dumbbells at your sides.

● Take a bold stride forward, far enough so that your front thigh ends up parallel to the floor with your knee over (not past) your toes. Quickly push back up to the starting position.

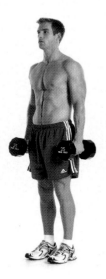

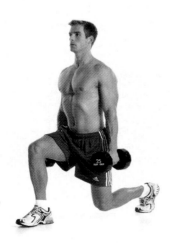

SUPERSET 3

SWISS BALL JACKKNIFE (Alternate: V-Up)

● Get into a pushup position, with the tops of your feet and your shins on the ball and your hands on the floor.

● Pull your knees close to your chest, letting the ball roll slightly forward. Keep your arms straight, and squeeze your abs hard at the top.

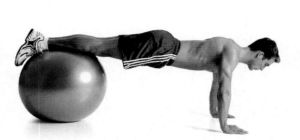

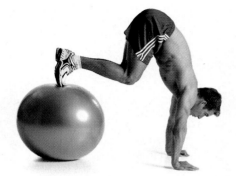

DIP (Alternate: Close-Grip Bench Press)

● Step onto the foot supports of a dip station, grabbing the ends of the handles with a neutral grip (thumb on opposite side of fingers, palms facing in). Jump up, and steady yourself. Start the movement with your arms straight but not locked, and your body perfectly still. Cross your legs behind you or leave them hanging straight down.

● Slowly lower yourself until your upper arms are parallel to the floor. (If possible, do this in front of a mirror; going lower is brutal to your shoulders.) Push back up to the starting position.

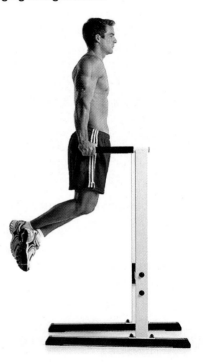 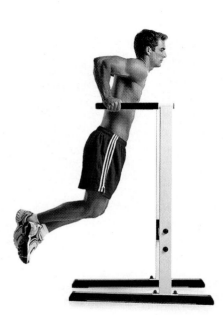

This workout series is adapted from *The Men's Health Home Workout Bible,* by Lou Schuler, with exercise programs by Michael Mejia, M.S., C.S.C.S. © 2002 by Rodale Inc. Available wherever books are sold.

Training

Tips

FIRST THINGS FIRST

If I want to lose a lot of body fat, do I have to do cardiovascular exercise first thing in the morning, on an empty stomach?

G.B., ERIE, PENNSYLVANIA

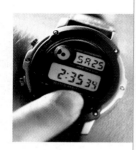

That's actually a bad idea. First, your body temperature is lowest in the morning, which means it takes much longer to warm up and get your muscles, joints, and nerves working together and protecting you from injury.

Second, your cortisol level is highest early in the day. Cortisol is a stress hormone that can signal your body to consume muscle for energy. So, in theory, morning exercise would have a muscle-wasting effect, like dropping your body into the middle of a marathon.

Finally, morning exercise proponents say you'll burn fat instead of carbohydrates when you work out before breakfast. That's a myth: Your body burns mostly fat while you sleep, so you have plenty of carbohydrate-derived fuel in the tank when you get up.

Exercise works best when your body most wants to do it. If that's in the morning, at least be sure to eat something first.

WHEY OR NAY?

What's the best protein supplement—whey or soy?

R.R., ORINDA, CALIFORNIA

Whey (animal protein) is superior to soy (plant protein) as a muscle builder. And Baylor University researchers found a way to make whey way better: Add casein, a protein found in cottage cheese and milk. When a group of 36 men with at least 6 weeks of weight training experience were given a

TIME IT RIGHT

Give Your Weight-Loss Effort a Lift

You already know your body has to burn calories to process and store food. But now researchers at the University of Nevada have found that lifting weights before you eat a high-carbohydrate meal increases the thermic effect on food. And "increasing your thermic effect can aid in weight loss," says John Young, Ph.D., the lead study author. When the researchers studied the impact of completing a 30-minute workout before a high-carb meal, they found that it increased the calorie-burning effect by 73 percent. Here's why: Working out lowers glycogen levels, which triggers your body to process more of your postworkout meal into new glycogen.

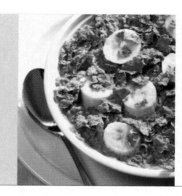

whey/casein mixture before their workouts, they built 50 percent more lean muscle mass over 10 weeks than men who took only whey. Casein slows down catabolism, a process in which your body breaks down muscle instead of fat for fuel. "When taken before a workout, casein may slow catabolism enough to help the body build more muscle," says study author Richard Kreider, Ph.D.

Q **I work out a lot. What vitamins should I take?**
L.S., ST. LOUIS, MISSOURI

A "Antioxidants are among the most important supplements when you're working out," says Shari Lieberman, Ph.D., C.N.S., F.A.C.N., author of *The Real Vitamin and Mineral Book*. They minimize muscle soreness, allowing you to do more exercise. Antioxidants counter the damaging effects of oxygen free radicals, which accumulate during exercise. If your muscles are iron, free radicals are rust. "They're the bad guys that speed up the aging process and lead to disease," says Earl Mindell, Ph.D., author

RECIPE

Muscle Chow

Here's one of *Men's Health* cover model Gregg Avedon's favorite postworkout meals for restoring energy and building muscle. The protein helps your muscles grow, while the complex carbohydrates restock the glycogen you've just burned off, providing energy for tomorrow's workout. Your muscles will look fuller because glycogen helps store water in your muscle cells.

Gregg's rule: Always take in protein and a small amount of unsaturated fat whenever you eat carbohydrates, to keep your metabolism consistent throughout the day.

Pasta contains about 7 grams of protein per serving, but this protein lacks essential amino acids. The low-fat cheese and edamame (green soybeans) make the protein usable for building muscle. The soybeans add healthy fat and fiber, so your blood glucose won't spike.

1 Tbsp each extra-virgin olive oil, chopped oregano, chopped basil, and chopped red pepper
1 c frozen shelled edamame
2 c whole-wheat pasta (like ziti or bow ties)
2 c broccoli florets
2 c cubed yellow squash
2 small zucchini, sliced
1 3½-oz package reduced-fat feta cheese, crumbled
1 Tbsp Parmesan cheese (optional)

Throw the olive oil, oregano, basil, red pepper, and edamame into a large pot of water, and bring to a boil. Add the pasta, broccoli, squash, and zucchini, and cook until the pasta is al dente. (Check the package for instructions.) Crumble the feta into a big bowl. Strain the cooked pasta until dripping (not dry), then dump it all in the bowl with the cheese and toss till it's mixed. Top with the Parmesan, if using. Makes three servings.

Per serving: 474 calories, 27 g protein, 68 g carbohydrates, 13 g fat, 13 g fiber, 544 mg sodium

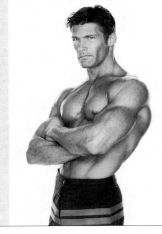

of the *Vitamin Bible*. Lieberman recommends this antioxidant arsenal for heavy exercisers:

Vitamin A: 5,000 to 25,000 international units (IU)

Vitamin C: 1 to 2 grams (1,000 to 2,000 milligrams)

Natural vitamin E with mixed tocopherols: 400 to 1,200 IU

Natural beta-carotene with mixed carotenoids: 11,000 to 25,000 IU

Selenium: 200 to 400 micrograms

WEIGHT LOSS SCAM

The High Price of Low-Carb

From beer to ice cream, everything's available in a low-carb version. But what are you really buying? Turns out many foods labeled "low-carb" contain about the same amounts of carbohydrates as their sugar-free equivalents, but often cost twice as much. See for yourself. Check the nutrition labels of low-carb products, and you'll find "net carbohydrates" listed. This is the number of so-called bad carbs that remain after you subtract fiber and sugar alcohols—two carbs that don't cause a spike in blood-sugar levels. While you may not find net carbs on sugar-free-food labels, they do list fiber and sugar alcohols, so you can calculate the net number. As you'll see, the only significant difference between a low-carb food and a sugar-free one is the price.

PRODUCT	NET CARBS	PRICE
4-pack low-carb meal-replacement shakes	1 g	$9.99
4-pack sugar-free meal-replacement shakes	1 g	$6.99
Low-carb protein bar	3 g	$2.60
Sugar-free protein bar	1 g	$0.97
10-oz jar low-carb fruit spread	2 g	$5.99
12.75-oz jar sugar-free fruit spread	5 g	$2.47
12-oz bottle low-carb pancake syrup	1 g	$4.99
12-oz bottle sugar-free pancake syrup	0 g	$1.99
3-oz bag low-carb jelly beans	3 g	$2.69
3.1-oz bag sugar-free jelly beans	4 g	$2.49
4-serving package low-carb ice cream	4 g	$4.89
4-serving package sugar-free ice cream	9 g	$5.49
2-serving package low-carb peanut-butter cups	1 g	$4.49
3.3-oz bag sugar-free peanut-butter cups	3 g	$1.99

GAINS AND LOSSES

Q **Is it possible to gain muscle and lose fat at the same time?**
S.G., LOS ALAMOS, NEW MEXICO

A Not really. If you're pretty lean and add weight, most of it will be muscle. But the heavier you are, the higher the percentage of fat you'll gain if you put on any pounds. That's why the most effective strategy, in my view, is to first lose the fat you want to lose, through strict diet and exercise, then up the calories to add more muscle. The easiest way: Cut carbohydrates on the way down, and add them on the way up.

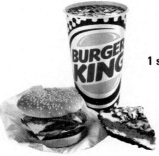

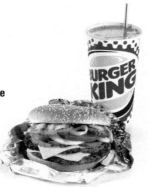

At Burger King

MEAL #1
1 Bacon Double
Cheeseburger
1 slice Hershey Sundae Pie
1 large Diet Coke

MEAL #2
1 Double Whopper
with Cheese
1 medium chocolate shake

TOTAL: 890 CALORIES,
38 G PROTEIN,
65 G CARBOHYDRATES,
52 G FAT (30 G SATURATED)

TOTAL: 1,940 CALORIES,
79 G PROTEIN,
142 G CARBOHYDRATES,
118 G FAT (57 G SATURATED)

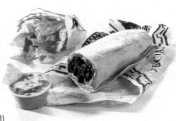

At Taco Bell

MEAL #1
3 Beef Hard Tacos
with everything

MEAL #2
1 Grilled Stuft Beef
Burrito with Nachos

TOTAL: 510 CALORIES,
27 G PROTEIN,
39 G CARBOHYDRATES,
30 G FAT (12 G SATURATED)

TOTAL: 1,080 CALORIES,
33 G PROTEIN,
108 G CARBOHYDRATES,
58 G FAT (16 G SATURATED)

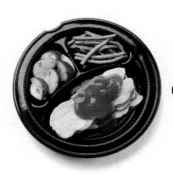

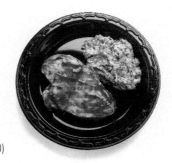

At Boston Market

MEAL #1
Skinless Rotisserie
Turkey Breast
Side of Chicken Gravy
Green Beans
Garlic Dill New Potatoes

MEAL #2
Grilled Barbecue
Chicken
Creamed Spinach

TOTAL: 385 CALORIES,
40 G PROTEIN,
36 G CARBOHYDRATES,
8 G FAT (3 G SATURATED)

TOTAL: 660 CALORIES,
50 G PROTEIN,
27 G CARBOHYDRATES,
39 G FAT (20 G SATURATED)

MASTER YOUR MUSCLES

Men have always had the attitude that bigger is better. We strive to get the bigger car, bigger house, bigger bank account. Our muscles are no different. We don't settle for small. And unlike a car or house or a guy's net worth, your muscles are always with you, a visible sign to everyone you meet that you're a man who makes big things happen.

This is where Big begins. The following pages are loaded with workouts, tips, shortcuts, and even secrets that will bulk up any guy looking for a big return on his exercise investment.

Since we're not big on wasting your time, we'll cut right to the chase. Grab some iron, and turn the page.

BY IAN KING, C.S.C.S., AND LOU SCHULER

Muscle Secrets

They lift and tell. The guys who wrote the book on getting bigger and stronger reveal 9 muscle secrets that will change your body

Your body has about 650 muscles. It doesn't matter that you only care about four or five of them. You need every one in order to perform the normal functions of everyday life—eating, breathing, walking, holding in your stomach at the beach.

Granted, you don't need to spend a lot of time thinking about most of your muscles. The 200 muscles involved in walking do the job whether you monitor them or not. You could try to impress your friends at parties by telling them the gluteus maximus is the body's strongest muscle, or that the latissimus dorsi (in your middle back) is the largest, or that a middle-ear muscle called the stapedius is the smallest. But it probably won't work, unless you have some really unusual friends. And muscle trivia can't capture the wonder of muscles themselves—the brilliance of coordinated muscles in motion, the magnificence of well-developed muscles in isolation.

We hope, in the following pages, to help you understand a little more about how your muscles work, and thus how to make them bigger, stronger, and more aesthetically pleasing (if you're into that sort of thing). You can accomplish all three, if you know what's going on beneath the surface.

Secret #1
MUSCLE FIBERS, LIKE CHILDREN, HAVE DIFFERENT ABILITIES

Your skeletal muscles—the ones you check out in the mirror—have two main types of fibers. Type I fibers, also called slow-twitch, are used mainly for endurance activities. Type II, or fast-twitch, begin to work when a task utilizes more than 25 percent of your maximum strength. A movement doesn't have to be "slow" for the slow-twitch fibers to take over; it just has to be an action that doesn't require much of your fast-twitch strength. And an effort doesn't have to be "fast" to call your fast-twitch fibers into play. A personal-record bench press is going to use every possible fast-twitch fiber (plus all the slow-twitchers, as we'll explain below), even though the bar probably isn't moving very fast.

Most people are thought to have a more or less equal mix of slow- and fast-twitch fibers. (Elite athletes are obvious exceptions—a gifted marathoner was probably born with more slow- than fast-twitch fibers, just as an Olympic-champion sprinter or NFL running back probably started life with

PEAK performance

Mix It Up for More Muscle

Most lifters vary their workouts after a month because they know muscles adapt to stress. But two recent studies at Arizona State University show that when and how you vary your workouts is what determines whether you improve strength or endurance. In the first study, men who changed to fewer repetitions using more weight at every workout gained 50 percent more strength on the bench press than those who made the same change to their workout routine every 4 weeks. In the second study, men who increased repetitions while decreasing weight once a month improved endurance. Improving endurance requires a gradual increase in volume, while strength responds to frequent changes, says Matthew Rhea, Ph.D., the lead study author.

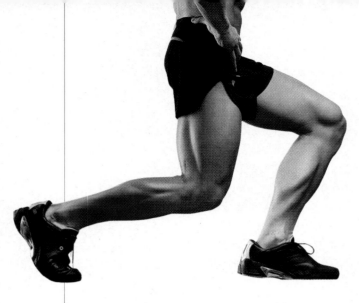

more fast-twitch fibers.) However, the fast-twitch fibers are twice as big as the slow ones, with the potential to get even bigger. Slow-twitch fibers can get bigger, too, although not to the same extent.

So one strategy comes immediately to mind. . . .

Secret #2
TO GROW LARGE, YOU MUST LIFT LARGE

When you begin a task, no matter if it's as simple as getting out of bed or as complex as swinging a golf club, your muscles operate on two basic principles of physiology:

1. The all-or-nothing principle states that either a muscle fiber gets into the action or it doesn't. (As Yoda said, long ago in a galaxy far away, "There is no try.") If it's in, it's all the way in. So when you get up to walk to the bathroom, incredibly enough, a small percentage of your muscle fibers are working as hard as they can to get you there. And,

more important, all the other fibers are inactive.

2. The size principle requires that the smallest muscle fibers get into a task first. If the task—a biceps curl, for example—requires less than 25 percent of your biceps' strength, then the slow-twitch fibers will handle it by themselves. When the weight exceeds 25 percent of their strength, the type II, fast-twitch fibers jump in. The closer you get to the limits of your strength, the more fast-twitch fibers get involved.

Here's why this is important: One of the most pervasive myths in the muscle world is that merely exhausting a muscle will bring all its fibers into play. So, in theory, if you did a lot of repetitions with a light weight, eventually your biggest type II fibers would help out because the smaller fibers would be too tired to lift the weight.

But the size principle tells you that the biggest fibers are the Mafia hit men of your body. They don't help the underlings collect money from deadbeats. They suit up only when the work calls for their special talents, and when no one else can be trusted to do the job right.

In other words, a guy who's trying to build as much muscle as possible must eventually work with weights that require something close to an all-out effort. Otherwise, the highest-threshold fibers would never spring into action. Moreover, the smaller fibers don't need any special high-repetition program of their own, since the size principle also says that if the big fibers are pushed to the max, the small ones are getting blasted, too.

Secret #3
YOU CAN SAVE YOUR BONES BY BUILDING YOUR MUSCLES

Many have tried to disparage the squat, framing it as an exercise that's brutal to back and knees. The charges never stick. Sure, the exercise can be tough on the knees, but no tougher than full-court basketball or other full-bore sports. And for guys with healthy backs and knees, the squat is among the best exercises for strength, mass, sports performance, and even long-term health. The heavy loads build muscle size and strength, along with bone density, and thicker bones will serve you well when you finally break into that 401(k). So you won't be the guy who fractures his hip and ends up in a nursing home, although you'll probably pay some visits to your nonsquatting friends.

Setup: (See photos below.) Set a bar in supports that are just below shoulder height, and load the weight plates. (Be conservative with these weights if you've never squatted before. There's a learning curve.) Grab the bar with your hands just outside your shoulders, then step under the bar and rest it on your back. When you pull your shoulder blades together in back, the bar will have a nice shelf to rest on. Lift the bar off the supports, and take a step back. Set your feet shoulder-width apart, bend your knees slightly, pull in your lower abs, squeeze your glutes, and set your head in line with your spine, keeping your eyes forward.

Descent: To begin the squat, bend your knees and hips simultaneously to lower your body. Squat as deeply as you can without allowing your trunk to move forward more than 45 degrees from vertical. Make sure your heels stay flat on the floor.

Ascent: Squeeze your glutes together, and push them forward to start the ascent, which should mirror the descent. Keep your knees the same distance apart (don't let them move in or out). Your hips and shoulders need to move at the same angle—if your hips come up faster, you increase your trunk angle and risk straining your lower back. At the top, keep a slight bend in your knees.

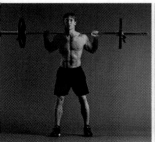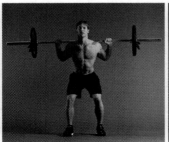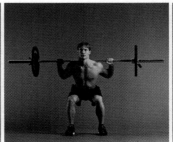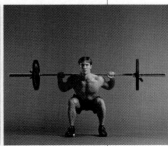

Secret #4
YOUR QUANTITY OF MUSCLE FIBERS IS SET AT BIRTH. THE QUALITY OF THOSE FIBERS IS UP TO YOU

On the day you were conceived, the gene gods made three decisions that you might want to quibble with as an adult, if you could:

1. Your maximum number of muscle fibers

2. Your percentages of fast- and slow-twitch fibers

3. The shapes of your muscles when fully developed

On the downside, unless you were born to anchor the 4x100 relay at the next Olympics, you can forget about ever reaching that goal. The athletes at the extremes—the fastest and strongest, the ones with the best-looking muscles, and the ones capable of the greatest endurance—were already at the extremes from the moment sperm swam headlong into egg.

The upside is that there's a lot of wiggle room in between. Few of us ever approach our full genetic potential. You probably will never be a freak, but with the right kind and amount of work, you can always be a little freakier than you are now.

The best way to do that is to learn to use your muscles' very own juice machine.

Secret #5
IF YOU WANT MORE MUSCLE, YOU NEED MORE TESTOSTERONE

Everyone has some testosterone—babies, little girls playing with tea sets, grandparents shuffling through the laxative aisle at CVS—but no one has hormonal increases from one year to the next like a maturing male. His level increases tenfold during puberty, starting sometime between ages 9 and 15, and he hits near-peak production in his late teens. From there, his testosterone level climbs slowly until about age 30, at which point he hits or passes a few other peaks.

His muscle mass will top out between the ages of 18 and 25, unless he intervenes with some barbell therapy. Sexual desire peaks in his early 30s. Sports performance, even among elite athletes, peaks in the late 20s and starts to decline in the early 30s.

None of this is inevitable, of course. Unless you're that elite athlete who's trained for his sport since before the short hairs sprouted, you probably have the potential to grow bigger and stronger than you've ever been. And that could also put a little of

PAINkiller

Is it normal for your shoulder to pop and crack when lifting weights?

Phil R., Enid, Oklahoma

No, any time your shoulder makes noises you'd hear from your cereal, you've got trouble. Either there's something structurally wrong in that shoulder—like bone spurs or damaged tendons in your rotator cuff—or there's something wrong with your lifting form. The shoulder is a complicated joint with lots of muscles, tendons, and ligaments. If you're hearing noises but not feeling pain, then your body might be giving you a warning sign of imminent injury, and you need to pay attention. If you're experiencing pain along with this noise, that's a big red flag. Stop what you're doing, and get it checked out. Shoulder injuries can last a lifetime.

that teenage explosiveness back into your sex life.

The testosterone/muscle mass link is pretty clear in general terms: The more you have of one, the more you get of the other. Strength training, while it doesn't necessarily make your testosterone level go up permanently, certainly makes it get a little jiggy in the short term. We know of four ways to create a temporary surge in your most important hormone.

1. Do exercises that employ the most muscle mass, such as squats, deadlifts, pullups, and dips. (Three of these four exercises appear on these pages.)

2. Use heavy weights, at least 85 percent of the maximum you can lift once on any given exercise.

3. Do a lot of work during your gym time—multiple exercises, multiple sets, multiple repetitions.

4. Keep rest periods fairly short—30 to 60 seconds.

Of course, you can't do all these things in the same workout. For example, when you work a lot of muscle mass with heavy weights, you can't do a high volume of exercise, nor can you work effectively with short rest periods. This is among the many reasons you should periodize your workouts, which is a polysyllabic way of saying change your workouts every few weeks, rather than do the same thing from now until the gene gods recall the merchandise.

Secret #6
GROWING MUSCLES NEED MORE THAN PROTEIN

The mythology surrounding protein and muscle building could fill a book, even though the science is fairly straightforward. Your muscles are made of protein (except the four-fifths that's water), so you have to eat protein to make them grow. You also have to eat protein to keep them from shrinking, which is why men trying to lose fat without sacrificing muscle do best when they build their diets around high-quality, muscle-friendly protein from lean meat, fish, eggs, poultry, and low-fat dairy products.

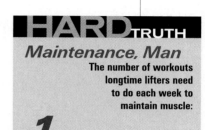

HARD TRUTH

Maintenance, Man

The number of workouts longtime lifters need to do each week to maintain muscle:

1

But if you're young, lean, and trying to gain solid weight, a lot of extra protein may not help as much as you think. Protein has qualities that help weight loss and may curtail weight gain. First, protein is metabolically expensive for your body to process. Your body burns about 20 percent of each protein calorie just digesting it. (It burns about 8 percent of carbohydrate and 2 percent of fat during digestion.)

Second, protein creates a high level of satiety, both during meals and between them. In other words, it makes you feel fuller faster and keeps you feeling full longer between meals. (This effect does wear off as you grow accustomed to a higher-protein diet, so it may not have an impact on long-term weight gain or weight loss.)

Finally, if you eat more protein than your body needs, it will learn to use the protein for energy. You want your body to burn carbohydrates and fat for energy, obviously, so a body that's relying on protein for energy is like a car that's using pieces of its engine for fuel.

The best weight gain strategy is to focus on calories first, protein second. You should make sure you're eating at least 2 grams (g) of protein per kilogram (kg) of muscle mass. A kilogram is 2.2 pounds, so a 160-pound guy weighs about 73 kg and should take in a minimum of 146 g of protein a day. But that's just 584 calories of protein, the amount you'd find in 15 ounces of chicken, two salmon fillets, or a 28-ounce steak. A protein-powder shake can amp up your totals, as well. If you need to eat more than 3,000 calories a day to gain weight, you'd better have some sweet potatoes with those steaks.

Secret #7
TO BUILD THE MUSCLE THAT COUNTS WHEN YOU NEED IT MOST, DO THE DEADLIFT

Ever watched a Strongman competition on TV? They start with large men picking something even larger up off the ground. That's a deadlift—the most basic and practical of all strength-building movements. Now, have you ever watched a Strongman competition with your wife or girlfriend? She'll notice something you probably

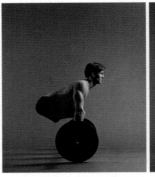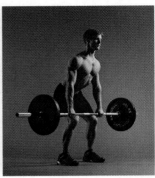

wouldn't: Not a single one of those guys has a flat ass. So pull up a barbell: You'll be able to perform everyday feats of strength— lifting a sleeping child or a dying TV—and you'll look a lot better when she follows you upstairs to the bedroom.

Setup: (See photos above and on next page.) Load a barbell, and roll it up to your shins. Stand with your feet shoulder-width apart. Position your shoulders over the bar as you grab it with an overhand grip, your hands just outside your knees. Keep your back in a straight line from head to pelvis. Finally, pull your shoulder blades together and down.

Just before the lift: Straighten your legs a bit to establish tension on the bar. Pull in your lower abs, and squeeze your glutes.

First pull, from floor to knees: Straighten your legs while keeping your trunk and hips at or near the same angle. The bar should stay in contact with your skin at all times.

Second pull, from knees to midthighs: Stand up, driving your hips forward. Finish upright, with your shoulder blades back and down and your lower back flat.

Lowering: No need to perfectly reverse the motion; just slide the bar down your

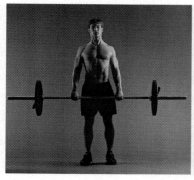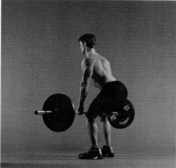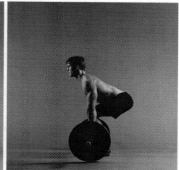

thighs and shins to the floor. Don't annoy your fellow lifters by dropping the bar.

Next repetition: Repeat the setup, letting go of the bar and regripping if necessary. You want perfect form on every repetition, and you won't get that if you bang out reps without stopping to set up properly before each lift. Remember, it's a deadlift. That means no momentum from one repetition to the next.

If you use perfect form, your lower back should give you no trouble. However, if you have preexisting back problems, your muscles may not fire properly for this exercise. Try the sumo deadlift instead. Set your feet wide apart, toes pointed slightly outward, and grip the bar overhand with your hands inside your knees. Your back will be more upright at the start, taking away some of the potential for strain.

Secret #8
IF YOU WANT BIG TRICEPS, DROP THE DUMBBELL AND LIFT YOURSELF

Beginners almost invariably hit their triceps with light weights, limited ranges of motion, and simple, easy exercises. Which is fine . . .

for beginners. For sizeaholics, the key to triceps development is lifting really, really heavy loads.

If you have time for just one triceps exercise, make it a dip. It's the big, basic movement that works all three parts of the muscle (thus the name "triceps"). And, because the bigger, stronger chest muscles are the prime movers—the ones that get your body moving from a dead-hang position—your triceps get to work against a much heavier load than they would in a triceps-isolating exercise.

How to dip: (See photos on next page.) Hoist yourself up on parallel bars with your torso perpendicular to the floor; you'll maintain this posture throughout the exercise. (Leaning forward will shift emphasis to your chest and shoulders.) Bend your knees, and cross your ankles. Slowly lower your body until your shoulder joints are below your elbows. (Most guys stop short of this position.) Push back up until your elbows are nearly straight but not locked.

Making progress: For most men, doing sets of dips with their own body weight is challenging enough. But when you reach a

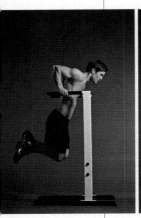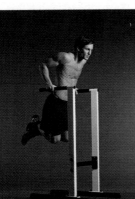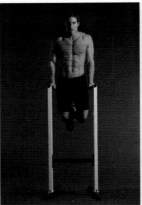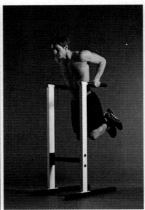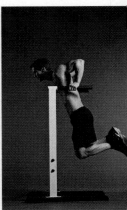

point at which you can do multiple sets of 10 dips, you want to add weight. The best way is to attach a weight plate or dumbbell to a rope or chain that's attached to a weight belt. Many gyms have belts specially designed for weighted dips and chinups. Another solution, especially if you work out at home, is to wear a backpack with weight plates inside it.

But the more weight you add, the more careful you have to be. Always lower yourself slowly—you don't ever want to pop down and up quickly on a weighted dip, unless you think you'll relish the feeling of your pectoral muscles detaching from your breastbone.

Precautions: Aside from the pec-tearing thing, you want to protect your shoulders. If you have preexisting shoulder problems, or feel pain there the first few times you try dips, you should skip dips.

A comparable but more shoulder-friendly exercise is the decline close-grip bench press, using a barbell or dumbbells held together.

Secret #9
IF SIZE IS YOUR GOAL, AVOID THE SHRINKING MAN'S EXERCISE

Running doesn't build muscle mass. If it did, marathoners would have legs like defensive linemen, and workers in Boston would have to repave the streets each year following the city's signature race. But running shrinks muscle fibers to make them more metabolically efficient, thereby saving the pavement.

You'd think you could get around this by lifting weights in addition to running, but your body negates that work through a mysterious "interference effect." Your type II fibers—the biggest ones—will still grow if you run and lift. But your type I fibers won't, and even though they're smaller than the type IIs, they probably comprise 50 percent of the muscle fibers in your body that have any growth potential.

Cut back on your running program, and you'll see growth in both your slow- and fast-twitch muscle fibers, and perhaps finally get your body to look the way you think it should.

Excerpted from *The Book of Muscle* (Rodale Inc., 2003), available at menshealth.com or wherever books are sold.

Get Sets, Grow

Gain strength and size with the right combination of sets and reps

You've been told to listen to your body, learn its idiosyncrasies, embrace it like a friend. Don't buy it. You can listen and learn, sure, but forget the friendly stuff. When it comes to muscle, you need to be less good buddy and more psychotic drill sergeant.

Keep your muscles off balance. When they get used to lifting a certain amount in a certain way (sound like your workout?), they stop growing. A training program that never changes also creates strength imbalances; that's unproductive and dangerous.

This doesn't mean you have to master the incline behind-the-back modified Slovenian triceps windmill. Just do your usual exercises, but use different combinations of sets and repetitions.

What follows is a guide to different kinds of sets and how they produce different results, from trainer Craig Ballantyne, C.S.C.S., owner of workoutmanuals.com. Plug this into your gym routine and see the surprised—and supersized—reaction you get from your muscles.

Straight Sets

What they are: The usual—a number of repetitions followed by a rest period, then by one or more sets of the same exercise.

Why they're useful: The rest periods and narrow focus of straight sets help add mass and build maximal strength. As long as you rest enough between sets (1 to 3 minutes), your muscle, or group of muscles, will work

hard two, three, even five times in a workout.

How to use them: The start of your workout is the best time to do straight sets, regardless of your experience level, Ballantyne says. Your energy and focus are high at the start, so it's the best time to execute difficult moves. Perform three straight sets of six to eight repetitions of a challenging exercise like the bench press, pullup, or squat; aim to do the same number of repetitions in each set, with either the same or increasing amounts of weight.

Supersets

What they are: A set of each of two different exercises performed back-to-back, without rest.

Why they're useful: Supersets save time and burn fat. You can multitask your muscles—for instance, working your chest and back in one superset, then the legs and shoulders in another. Lifting heavy weights in a short time period increases the rate at which your body breaks down and rebuilds protein. This metabolism boost lasts for hours after you've finished lifting.

How to use them: Insert a superset at any time in your workout. To involve the most muscles, pair compound exercises—moves that work multiple muscles across multiple joints. For example, combine a chest press with a row, or a shoulder press with a deadlift. To save more time, pair noncompeting muscle groups, such as your deltoids and glutes. One muscle group is able to recover while the other works, so you can repeat the set without resting as long.

Trisets

What they are: Three different exercises performed one after another, without any rest in between.

Why they're useful: Trisets save time and raise metabolism. A single triset can be a total-body workout in itself.

How to use them: Trisets are a good workout for at home (or in an empty gym), because you need to monopolize equipment for three exercises. Do basic exercises that hit different body parts—like bench presses, squats, and chinups. Perform a warmup set using 50 percent of the weight you usually use in each exercise. Then repeat the triset two or three times, using weights that allow you to perform eight repetitions per set. Rest 1 to 3 minutes after each triset.

Drop Sets

What they are: Three or four sets of one exercise performed without rest, using a lighter weight for each successive set. Also called descending sets or strip sets.

Why they're useful: Drop sets are a great quick workout, fatiguing your muscles in a short time, getting your heart going, and giving you an impressive postworkout pump as your muscles fill with blood.

How to use them: Use drop sets when you're pressed for time. Don't do them more than three times a week; you'll get so tired that you won't be able to accomplish much

else. Start with a warmup, using 50 percent of the weight you expect to use in your first set. Now use the heaviest weight you'd use for eight repetitions of that exercise to perform as many repetitions as you can. Drop 10 to 20 percent of the weight, and go again. Continue to reduce the weight and go again, always trying to complete the same number of repetitions (even though you won't) until your muscles fail.

Circuit Sets

What they are: A series of exercises (usually six) that you complete one after another without rest, though you can do some cardiovascular work (such as jumping rope) between exercises.

Why they're useful: When you use weights, circuits can be a great total-body workout. But they're most valuable without weights as a warmup of the nervous system, joints, and muscles, Ballantyne says. Because a circuit stresses the entire body, it's more effective than a treadmill jog, which primes only your lower body.

How to use them: You'll annoy the other guys at the gym if you do an entire workout based on circuits, because you'll monopolize so many pieces of equipment. But one circuit is quick and effective. If you're using it as a warmup, you need only your body weight or a barbell (see "Combo-Platter Workout" on page 58). Or use just a pair of dumbbells and circuit-train at home where you won't annoy anyone.

Combo-Platter Workout

This full-body workout from trainer Craig Ballantyne runs the gamut of sets. It focuses on two often-neglected areas: the upper back and the "posterior chain"—the hamstrings, glutes, and lower back. The posterior chain gives you power and speed in sports.

Warmup Circuit

This is an all-purpose warmup for any strength-training workout. All you need is a barbell. Do eight repetitions of each exercise, and repeat the circuit twice.

Squat (body weight only)

Pushup (body weight only)

Reverse Lunge (body weight only)

Barbell Row (bar only)

Diagonal Lunge (body weight only)

Straight Sets

Perform three sets of six repetitions. Rest for 2 to 3 minutes after each set.

Sumo Squat Stand with your feet 6 inches more than shoulder-width apart, toes slightly turned out. Hold a dumbbell between your legs, with both hands under the top of the dumbbell. Keep your arms against your body.

Squat down until the dumbbell touches the floor, pause, then return to the starting position.

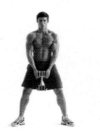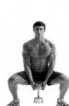

Superset #1

Do eight repetitions of each exercise without resting between the two exercises. Complete three supersets, resting for 1 minute after each.

Dumbbell Chest Press Lie on a bench, holding a pair of dumbbells directly over your chest with straight arms and an overhand grip (palms facing away from you). Keep your feet flat on the floor and angled to the sides for better balance.

Next, bend your arms to lower the dumbbells to the outsides of your chest, pause, then push the weights back up to the starting position.

Chinup Grab a chinup bar with an underhand grip—that is, with your palms facing you. Your hands should be slightly more than shoulder-width apart.

Keeping your head, shoulders, hips, and knees

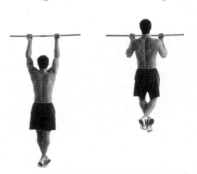

perfectly aligned, pull your chest to the bar, pause for a second, then lower yourself until your arms are straight again. To keep the tension on your back, resist locking your elbows.

Superset #2

Do 12 repetitions of each move with no rest. Rest 1 minute before repeating the superset. Complete three supersets.

Barbell Row Hold a barbell with an overhand grip, and stand with your knees slightly bent. Bend at the hips until your torso is almost parallel to the floor. Your arms should hang straight down.

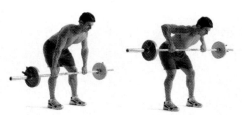

Pull the bar up until it's even with your lower rib cage. Pause, then lower the bar to the starting position.

Cable Lift Attach a stirrup handle to a low-pulley cable, and stand with your left foot toward the weight stack. Bend your knees and push your hips back to lower yourself into a squat. Reach across your body with straight arms, and grab the handle.

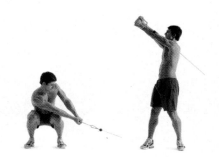

Keeping your abs tight and elbows locked, stand up and rotate your torso, bringing the handle above your opposite shoulder. Then slowly return to the squat position. After six repetitions, turn around and repeat the move with your right foot next to the stack.

Drop Sets

Do four sets of as many repetitions as possible, beginning with the most weight you can lift eight times and removing 10 to 20 percent of the weight after each set.

Lying Triceps Extension Lie on a bench, holding an EZ-curl bar with an overhand, shoulder-width grip. Hold the bar at arm's length over your forehead.

Keeping your upper arms in the same position throughout the move, bend at the elbows to lower the bar to the top of your forehead. Pause, then push the weight back up.

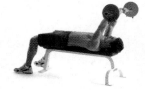
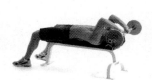

BY MARY CHRIST

Man and Machine

In the land of the free weight, the boost you can get from exercise machines is even more liberating

The typical hard-core lifter looks at weight machines and thinks: worthless. But that's not fair. The problem isn't with the machines; it's with the lifters.

Most men—if they use a machine—don't venture beyond the faded directions that were slapped on in the factory. Trouble is, a machine exercise circuit repeated day after day, year after year, is about as challenging as the workout routine of a fit 60-year-old woman.

Exercise variety is the path to better and faster muscle and strength gains—which is why serious lifters head for the free-weight room, where the iron isn't attached to contraptions and the variations are endless.

We offer a third option: new operating instructions. We'll show you how to make weight machines work better for you. You can use these strategies as training tools in your free-weight routine or to add juice to your tired machine workout. The end result: more muscle.

CHANGE YOUR BODY POSITION

Most machines have a fixed path of motion, meaning your first lift and your tenth are identical, says Alwyn Cosgrove, C.S.C.S., owner of Results Fitness in Santa Clarita, California. This can lead to "pattern overload syndrome," similar to carpal tunnel syndrome. You need to challenge your muscles from a variety of angles.

The Benefit: You'll build bigger muscles and avoid overload syndrome.

- When using "sit-down" machines such as the leg extension and seated chest press, adjust the seat position by an inch, up or down, between sets.

- On the leg-press and squat machines, place your feet farther apart or closer together.

- On machines that have multiple handles—the shoulder-press and row machines, for example—alternate your grip between palms facing forward and palms facing each other.

DON'T BRACE YOURSELF

Imagine that there's wet paint on the support pads of the machine, says Gunnar Peterson, C.S.C.S., a trainer in Beverly Hills, California.

The Benefit: You'll strengthen your core muscles for sports. Three examples:

- Lat pulldowns—Don't always put your knees under the roller pads.

- Leg extensions—Sit upright on the seat without using the back support.

- Hip extensions and rows—Avoid bracing your upper body on the chest pad.

DO SINGLE-ARM NEGATIVES

This means overloading your muscles during the eccentric—the lowering—portion of the lift. Choose a weight that's about 60 percent of the amount you can lift five times, and push the weight up normally.

At the top of the move, pause, then remove one arm from the handle and lower the weight as slowly as you can. Do four sets of five repetitions, switching arms each set.

The Benefit: This can lead to greater muscle growth than you get from conventional lifting. But limit it to once a week, says Cosgrove. Heavy eccentric training causes more muscle damage than normal lifting, so your muscles need longer to recover.

EXTEND YOUR SETS

Try this on biceps and triceps machines that have separate handles for each hand. Choose a heavy weight that you can lift only six to eight times with one arm. When you can't perform one more repetition, grab the other handle with your opposite arm—so you're using both arms to lift the weight—and do eight to 10 more repetitions.

The Benefit: Greater growth, because you'll exhaust the muscle fibers in the first

Faulty Equipment

Avoid these weight machines

True, machines help you avoid dropping a bar or dumbbell. But they're not always safe. "Some are outright dangerous," says Gary Guerrero, P.T., A.T.C., director of the U.S. Athletic Training Center in New York City. Here are three you should skip:

Standing-Calf-Raise Machine

Why it's bad: Most men can't handle a substantial amount of weight—often more than they

can squat—when doing this exercise because of the small range of motion of the calf raise. This adds up to a lot of unnecessary spinal compression, which can lead to severe back problems.

Smith Machine (for squats)

Why it's bad: The path the bar follows doesn't allow for proper spinal mechanics, which can place excessive stress on the lower back. That's because the natural movement of your body

during a squat is an arc, not straight up and down. Stick with the free-weight version.

Pec Deck

Why it's bad: It forces you to abduct your upper arm horizontally—that is, move it away from your body while holding it parallel to the floor—while rotating it backward against a heavy weight. This places tremendous stress on the front portion of your deltoid, which can lead to nerve injuries.

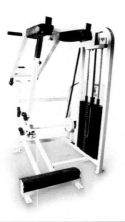

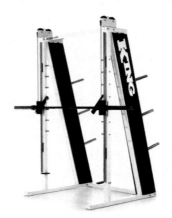

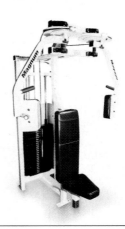

arm, says Tim Kuebler, C.S.C.S., a trainer in Kansas City, Missouri. Do four sets, alternating the arm you start with each time, every 4 days.

Or try combining a biceps and triceps workout by alternating exercises and arms, so that you do a right-arm curl, left-arm extension, left-arm curl, and right-arm extension. Rest for 60 seconds, then repeat one time.

COMPENSATE FOR POOR DESIGN

When using the seated-squat machine, place a rolled-up towel under the arch in your lower back. The change in posture creates a line of motion that's more consistent with the way you naturally squat, allowing your lower back and hips to move slightly behind your heels.

The Benefit: It reduces your risk of injury and better trains your muscles for the way they'll be used in real life, says Cosgrove.

FINISH WITH DROP SETS

On your last set of an exercise (free weight or machine), perform the same move on a "selectorized" machine such as Nautilus, Universal, or Cybex. Start with the most weight you can lift six to eight times, and do as many repetitions as possible. Immediately drop the weight by 20 percent and do six to eight more repetitions, then drop the weight by 20 percent again and do a final six- to eight-repetition set.

The Benefit: Your muscles will be forced to work harder than ever before and you'll gain strength, says Peterson.

COMBINE CABLES WITH DUMBBELLS

By attaching cables to your wrists when doing the dumbbell bench press, you'll add horizontal resistance to the exercise.

The Benefit: "It forces your muscles to work against both vertical and horizontal resistance," says Michael Mejia, C.S.C.S., *Men's Health* exercise advisor. Here's how: Put a weight bench in the center of a cable station, perpendicular to the machine. Select fairly light weights on both weight stacks. Fasten a pair of ankle straps to your wrists, and hook the straps to the low pulley of the cable station. Grab a pair of dumbbells (have them handy!) that are half the weight you'd usually use, lie on the bench, and hold the dumbbells at the sides of your chest. Perform a standard dumbbell press by pushing the dumbbells up and in, until your arms are straight and the dumbbells are almost touching.

PAINkiller

I hurt my right shoulder on my gym's shoulder-press machine. When I lift my arm, it feels as if something's pinching inside the socket. Now what?

First, promise that you'll never go near a shoulder-press machine again. Shoulder-press machines suck because they use a locked-in range of motion, which may be unnatural for your shoulder joints, and because most of them force both arms to lift on the same trajectory, which arms rarely do naturally.

Barbells can create the same problems, especially when you press them up from behind your neck. So dumbbells are the best for fragile shoulders.

The touchdown shoulder press is nearly injury-proof. Hold two dumbbells at shoulder level with your palms facing each other, then press them up, as if you were signaling a touchdown. It's a great movement for preventing and recovering from shoulder injury.

BY ADAM CAMPBELL

Muscle Camp

Attend six of the best muscle-building camps— right here, right now—and learn new tricks from world-class weight-lifting experts

Imagine if you could step into the pages of this book and get cutting-edge training advice, interactively, with VIP access to the top trainers in the world. You ask questions; they share secrets.

Turns out you can. Or come pretty close, anyway, without the *Weird Science* trip. Your viable alternative: Step into a muscle camp. These are places where guys can learn how to get bigger, stronger, faster, and leaner, from the experts who know how to do it best. It's like an investor getting a scoop on the next Greenspan decision. The effect on your muscle portfolio: immediate gains, with unlimited growth potential.

We found six camps that will accelerate your knowledge—and your results—in just a weekend. On the next few pages, you'll find our favorite moves from each. Try them—then make a reservation. There's always room for more muscle.

The Westside Deadlift

Set a new personal record in the deadlift by revising your form. Stand in front of a loaded barbell, and roll it toward your shins until it's directly under the front of your thighs. Squat down and grab the bar with a shoulder-width, overhand grip. Keep your back naturally arched throughout the entire move, but allow your shoulders to round forward. Before you lift the weight, make sure your shoulders are positioned behind the bar.

Now stand with the bar, thrusting your

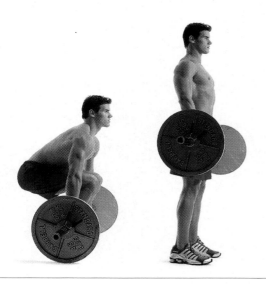

hips forward and pulling backward with your upper body (as if you were falling back). Lower the bar to the floor, release your grip, and stand up. Rest for 10 seconds, then position yourself again and repeat. Resting ensures that you put the same concentration on technique into each lift, and it trains "starting strength," the key to deadlifting heavy weights.

The camp: *Westside Barbell,* Columbus, Ohio. This is the place if your goal is to build pure strength in the bench press, squat, and deadlift. "Past attendees have added as much as 150 pounds to their squats and deadlifts, and 75 pounds to their bench presses, in the first year after taking our seminar," says Dave Tate, a powerlifter (he squats 740 pounds) and seminar instructor.

Sign up: For camp dates and registration information, visit elitefitnesssystems.com. Or learn at home with the 6-hour *Westside Seminar* video set ($135).

The Swiss Ball Chest Fly

This unique move will build your chest without weights. Place two Swiss balls next to each other, bend your elbows, and brace a forearm on each. Straighten the rest of your body so that you're in a pushup position, your body forming a straight line from your shoulders to your ankles.

Using your forearms, roll the balls out and away from your body—one to your right and one to your left—until your upper arms are in line with your shoulders. Pause, then return to the starting position by pulling the balls back together.

The camp: *The C.H.E.K Institute,* Encinitas, California. You'll learn how to incorporate Swiss ball training techniques into your weight workout, shore up weak spots, and create a more "functional" program.

"Training in an unstable environment transfers better to real-life activities," says owner Paul Chek.

Sign up: Seminars are available at the institute and other locations across the United States. Go to www.chekinstitute.com for reservations, books, and videos.

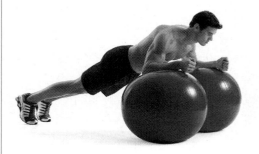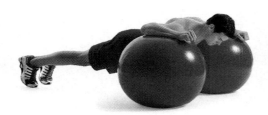

No Equipment, No Problem

Work your body without weights

You live in the real world; you're going to miss some workouts. But when there's no equipment at hand, you can rely on a technique from trainer Alwyn Cosgrove, C.S.C.S., called isoexplosive training. You'll use only your body weight to maintain muscle—whether you're on the road, stuck in the office, or just unable to find your dumbbells.

To eliminate the elasticity in your muscles, hold the "down" position of each exercise for 4 seconds. So when you explode upward, your muscle fibers will be forced to work maximally, without weights. For a quick full-body workout, simply try these versions of the pushup and squat. Do four or five sets of six to eight repetitions, alternating between exercises and resting 30 seconds between sets.

Isoexplosive Pushup Get into pushup position, hands slightly wider than and in line with your shoulders. Your body should form a straight line from your shoulders to your ankles. Keep your back flat, and lower your body until your upper arms are lower than your elbows. Pause, holding the "down" position for 4 seconds. Then forcefully thrust yourself upward as high as you can, so that your hands leave the floor. Catch yourself, and repeat.

Isoexplosive Squat Stand with your knees slightly bent and your feet shoulder-width apart. Slowly lower your body as if you were sitting back into a chair, keeping your back in its natural alignment, until the fronts of your thighs are parallel to the floor or lower. Pause, holding the "down" position for 4 seconds. Jump as high as you can, then repeat.

The Staley Curl

This modified curl strengthens you at the weak point in the biceps curl, which will allow you to use heavier weights when you return to regular curls; it could add an inch to your arms in 8 weeks. Set the pins in a power rack at about elbow level. Grab a barbell with an underhand grip, your hands as far apart as comfortable. Stand in front of the pins, holding the bar at arm's length in front of your thighs, your knees slightly bent and your feet shoulder-width apart.

Without moving your upper arms, curl the bar up so that it makes contact with the bottoms of the pins. Push up against the pins as hard as possible for 3 to 6 seconds, then return to the starting position. Repeat until you can no longer keep contact for 3 seconds. If you can't maintain contact for 3 seconds at the outset, use less weight.

The camp: *Staley Training Systems,* Las Vegas. Director Charles Staley specializes in training to build more muscle in less time—

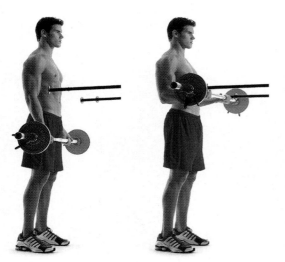

the perfect system for any guy with a packed schedule. Plus, you'll learn unconventional training methods designed to help you break through plateaus of muscle size and strength.

Sign up: For camp dates, books, or registration for Staley's private consultation group, go to staleytrainingsystems.com.

The Partial Co-Contraction Lunge

This basic lunge variation will be challenging for even the most battle-scarred gym veteran. Stand with your feet hip-width apart. Step forward with your nondominant leg (your left if you're right-handed), and lower your body until your front knee is bent 90 degrees and your back knee is touching the floor. Your front lower leg should be perpendicular to the floor, and your torso should remain upright. Place one hand on the vastus medialis—the teardrop muscle above the inside of your knee—of your front leg, and your other hand on the glute of the same leg. Raise your back knee 1 inch off the floor until you feel your vastus medialis and glute contract. That's the starting position.

Slowly raise yourself by straightening both legs simultaneously. The moment you lose maximal tension on either muscle, pause for 1 second, then slowly return to the starting position. When you finish your repetitions, switch legs.

The camp: *Results Fitness Training,* Santa Clarita, California. The name says it all. "Our typical client loses 30 to 35 pounds of fat in about 12 weeks," says owner Alwyn Cosgrove, C.S.C.S., a monthly contributor

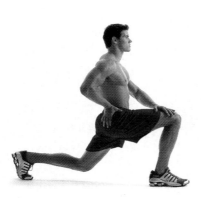
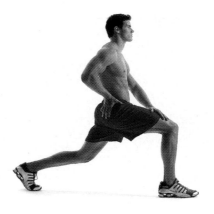

to *Men's Health* who trains athletes, models, and regular guys. His simple techniques can lead to dramatic results in fat loss, strength gain, muscle building, and performance.

Sign up: The private gym runs seminars for individuals and small groups. Go to results-fitness.com or call (661) 799-7900 for details.

The Burner

This move strengthens your abdominals at their weakest angle—a key to improving sports performance—while reducing your risk of knee injuries. Grab a dumbbell in your right hand with an overhand grip, and hold it at arm's length in front of your right thigh. Stand on your left leg, holding your right foot at least a few inches off the floor.

Reach down, and touch the dumbbell to the floor on the outside of your left foot by leaning forward and twisting your torso to the left.

Stand up, and reach behind your right shoulder with the dumbbell as you bend your left knee and twist to your right, keeping your right arm nearly straight. Pause, then lean forward and repeat.

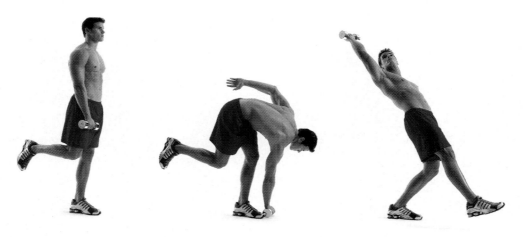

The camp: *The Competitive Athlete Training Zone (CATZ),* Pasadena, California. The staff has worked with recreational and professional athletes—including Oscar de la Hoya—from ages 9 to 66 for 10 years. "You'll learn how to improve speed, agility, power, strength, and mobility, all crucial elements of sports performance," says Jim Liston, C.S.C.S., owner of CATZ and the strength and conditioning coach for the Los Angeles Galaxy professional soccer team.

Sign up: The camp takes place at the Rose Bowl on weekends in July and August. For registration and information, go to catzsports.com.

The Turkish Getup

Use this long-forgotten exercise for fat loss and conditioning by performing multiple sets of low repetitions (no more than five per arm). As you improve, add more sets before adding more weight. Grab a kettlebell ($85 to $150 at russiankettlebell.com) or a dumbbell, and lie on the floor on your back, with your legs straight. Hold the kettlebell in your right hand directly above your chest, your arm straight and elbow locked.

From here, the move is simple: Stand up. Just three rules: Go slowly, never unlock your elbow, and keep the kettlebell above you at all times. So you'll probably roll onto your side, push yourself up with your free arm, then move to one knee, then stand upright, holding the kettlebell over your head. Reverse the movement, using the same rules. That's one repetition. (Switch arms each repetition.)

The camp: *Pavel Tsatsouline's Kettlebell Challenge Workshop,* Minneapolis, Minnesota. Tsatsouline, a former Soviet special-forces instructor, teaches you how to use kettlebells to build muscle and strength, and melt fat.

Sign up: Register and find books at russiankettlebell.com.

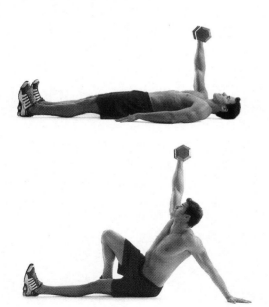
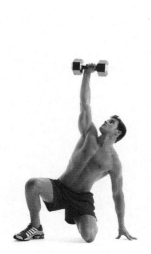
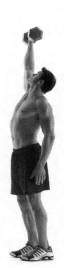

THE WORKOUT

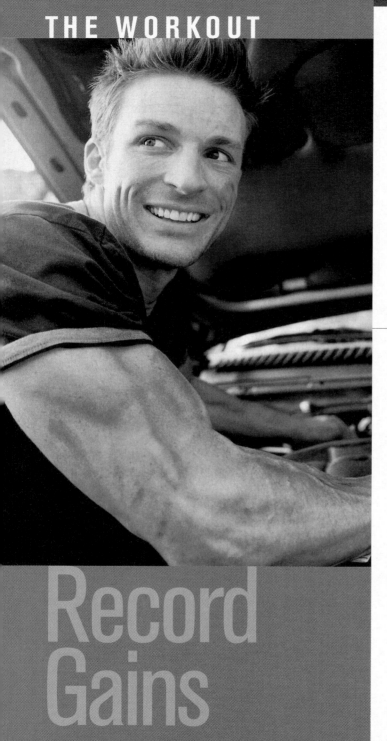

Record Gains

Lift more than ever with our maximum-strength plan

You invest your time and effort slinging iron at the gym or in your basement, and like any savvy businessman, you want to see a return on that investment. With this ultimate strength-building program, you'll experience record gains in just 4 weeks. Of course, you may need to invest in some larger shirts to accommodate those growing muscles, but hey, that's a price worth paying. Right?

Instructions

Most of the exercises in this workout are the same for both beginner and advanced lifters. The few exceptions are clearly labeled beginner or advanced. Choose the beginner level if you have less than a year of strength-training experience, or if you're coming back from a layoff of longer than 4 months. Choose the intermediate/advanced program if you've worked out consistently for the past year or longer.

If you belong to a gym, you can do the exercises exactly as shown here. Or, if you prefer, you can replace machine exercises with the barbell or dumbbell versions, or use dumbbells in place of the barbell.

BY MICHAEL MEJIA, C.S.C.S.

Alternate between workout A and workout B, doing one every 4 or 5 days, and perform the core workout (exercises that focus on your core, assistance, and stabilizer muscles) on 1 of the days in between. So you might do workout A on Monday, the core workout on Wednesday, workout B on Friday, and workout A again on Tuesday. For each exercise in workout A and workout B, perform five sets using a wave loading method, in which you alternate between three repetitions with a weight you can lift at most four times, and six repetitions with a weight you can lift at most seven times. So you'll do three repetitions in your first set, six repetitions in your second set, three repetitions in your third set, and so on. Rest for 3 minutes after each set. For each exercise in the core workout, do two or three sets of eight to 12 repetitions, with 60 seconds of rest after each set.

Alternate between workout A and workout B, doing one every 4 or 5 days, and perform the core workout (exercises that focus on your core, assistance, and stabilizer muscles) on 1 or 2 of the days in between. So you might do workout A on Monday, the core workout on Tuesday and Thursday, workout B on Saturday, the core workout again on Monday, and workout A again on Wednesday. For each exercise in workout A and workout B, perform six sets using a wave loading method, in which you perform four repetitions with a weight you can lift at most five times in the first set, three repetitions with a weight you can lift at most four times in the second set, and two repetitions with a weight you can lift at most three times in the third set, then repeat the cycle for your last three sets. Rest 3 minutes after each set. For each exercise in the core workout, do two or three sets of eight to 12 repetitions, with 60 seconds of rest after each set.

BARBELL DEADLIFT

● Load a barbell, and set it on the floor. Squat in front of it with your feet shoulder-width apart. Grab it overhand with your hands just outside your legs, your shoulders over or just behind the bar, your arms straight, and your back flat or slightly arched. (Your exact position depends on your unique biomechanics.)

● Simple as it sounds, all you really do is stand up. The key is to push with your heels and pull the weight to your body as you stand. Pause with the weight (don't lean back), then slowly return to the starting position. Pause with the weight on the floor, and reset your body over the bar.

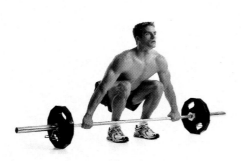
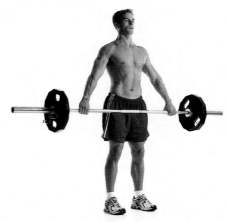

BARBELL BENCH PRESS

● Lie on a bench with your head, torso, and hips pressed against it and your feet spread wide and flat on the floor. Grab the barbell with a full (thumbs wrapped around the bar) overhand grip. Place your hands slightly wider than shoulder-width apart, remove the bar from the uprights, and hold it with straight arms over your collarbone. Pull your shoulder blades together in back.

● Lower the bar, slowly and in control, to just above your nipples. Then press it up and just slightly back, so it finishes above your collarbone again. Stop just short of locking your elbows, and keep your shoulder blades pulled back.

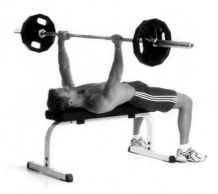
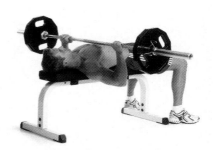

PULLUP/BEGINNER

● Grab a chinning bar with an overhand grip slightly wider than shoulder-width, and hang.

● Pull your chin above the bar, hold for a second or two, and lower your body with control.

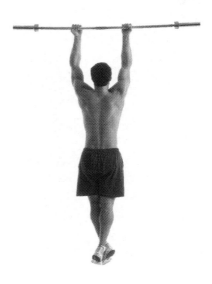

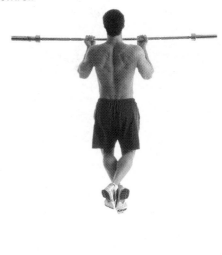

WEIGHTED PULLUP/ADVANCED

● Wearing a weighted belt, grab a chinning bar with an overhand grip slightly wider than shoulder-width, and hang.

● Pull your chin above the bar, hold for a second or two, and lower your body with control.

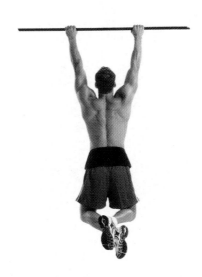

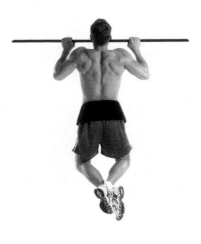

STANDING BARBELL CURL

● Grab the barbell with a full, underhand grip that's just wider than shoulder-width, and stand holding the bar at arm's length in front of your thighs. Set your feet shoulder-width apart, with your knees slightly bent, your back straight, and your abs pulled in.

● Without leaning back, curl the bar up toward your shoulders. When it's 6 inches from your shoulders, pause, and squeeze your biceps hard for a second or two. Then slowly return to the starting position.

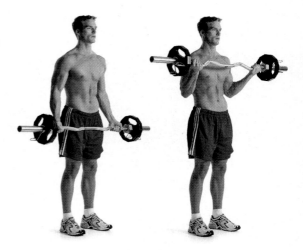

BARBELL SQUAT

● Set your barbell on the squat supports, so you have to bend your knees slightly to step under it and set it on your shoulders. (You don't want to have to lift it up to the supports at the end of a set—you may not be able to

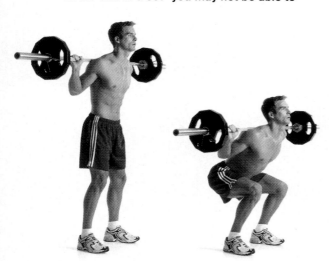

reach them.) Position yourself under the bar, so it rests on the backs of your shoulders and your trapezius, not your neck. (When you pull your shoulder blades back, your traps should form a nice shelf for the bar. It shouldn't hurt at all; if it does, it's a sure sign you're doing something wrong.) Hold the bar with a wide, overhand grip, straighten your legs to lift it off the rack, step back, and set your feet shoulder-width apart with your knees slightly bent and your lower back in its naturally arched position.

● Initiating the descent at the hips, not the knees, lower yourself as though sitting in a chair behind you. Stop when the tops of your thighs are parallel to the floor, pause, then push back up to the starting position. Your knees should stay in line with your feet throughout the movement; they shouldn't splay out or pinch in.

STANDING DUMBBELL SHOULDER PRESS

● Grab two dumbbells, and stand with your feet shoulder-width apart. Hold the weights with an overhand grip above each shoulder, in line with your jaws.

● Press the dumbbells straight up (not up and in). Pause, then slowly return to the starting position without letting the weights rest on your shoulders.

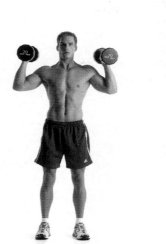 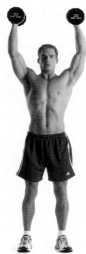

BARBELL BENT-OVER ROW

● Stand with your feet shoulder-width apart and your knees bent at 15 to 30 degrees. Keep your torso straight, with a slight arch in your back as you lean forward at the hips. Try to get your torso close to parallel to the floor. Grab the barbell off the floor with a false (thumbs in line with the rest of your fingers) overhand grip that's slightly wider than shoulder width. Let the bar hang at arm's length in front of you.

● Retract your shoulder blades to start pulling the bar up to the lower part of your sternum (breastbone). (Imagine that your arms are just along for the ride; otherwise, you'll use them as the prime movers and get less of a workout for your middle-back muscles.) Pause at the top, with your chest sticking out toward the bar. Slowly return to the starting position. Try to keep your torso in the same position throughout the movement. (That's the purpose of the bent knees—they provide the suspension your torso needs to remain steady.)

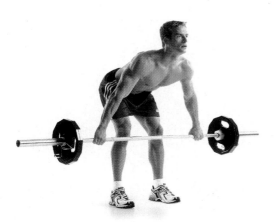 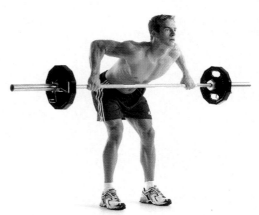

EZ-CURL-BAR FRENCH PRESS

● Grab the bar with a full, overhand grip that's just narrower than shoulder width. Sitting on the edge of a bench, hold the bar over your head with your arms straight but your elbows unlocked. Your upper arms should be just outside your ears.

● Bend your elbows, and slowly lower the bar toward the back of your neck. Stop when your forearms are just past parallel to the floor. Pause, then press back up to the starting position. Keep your upper arms in the same position throughout the exercise.

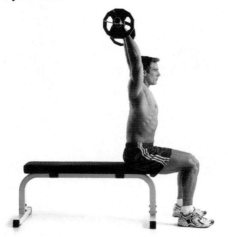

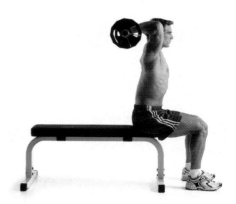

CORE WORKOUT

INCLINE REVERSE CRUNCH/BEGINNER

● Lie on an incline bench set at a 45-degree angle, so that your torso and buttocks are on the bench and your legs hang off. Using your abdominal muscles, hold your feet off the floor, keeping your knees slightly bent. To keep your body securely in place throughout the move, reach around and hold onto the bench supports.

● Use your abdominal muscles to crunch your pelvis toward your rib cage. Your tailbone should rise a few inches off the bench as your knees move toward your chin. Pause, then slowly return to the starting position.

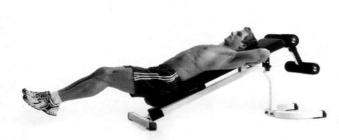

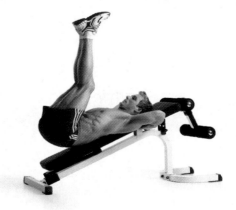

HANGING LEG RAISE/ADVANCED

● Grab a chinup bar with an overhead grip, and hang with your knees slightly bent.

● Use the muscles of your lower abs to pull your hips up as you curl them toward your chest. Lift your knees as close to your chest as possible, rounding your lower back at the top. Pause, and feel the contraction in your lower abdominal muscles. Then return to the starting position.

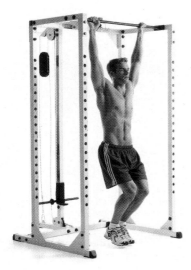

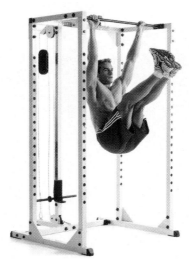

WEIGHTED RUSSIAN TWIST/BEGINNER

● Sitting on the floor with your knees bent and your feet flat, hold a light weight plate with your arms extended straight out in front of you. Lean back until your torso is at a 60- to 75-degree angle from the floor. Pull your belly in.

● Twist your torso as far as you can to one side and then to the other to complete the rep.

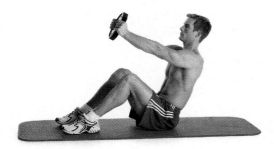

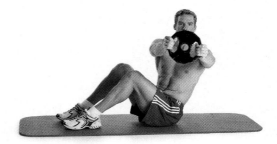

SWISS BALL RUSSIAN TWIST/ADVANCED

● Do the exercise while sitting on a Swiss ball instead of on the floor. Start in a regular crunch position on the ball. Lift your shoulders so they clear the ball.

● With your arms extended out in front, rotate from side to side, as in the standard Russian twist. Your hips and legs may shift a bit because of the ball's instability, and you won't be able to lean back as you did on the floor.

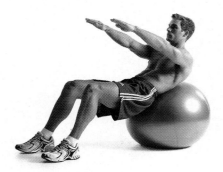 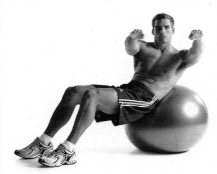

DUMBBELL CALF JUMP

● Holding a pair of dumbbells, bend your knees and squat straight down until your thighs are halfway to parallel to the floor (in a quarter-squat).

● Quickly and explosively jump into the air as high as possible, concentrating on pushing off with your calves rather than with the larger hamstrings or quadriceps. As you land, immediately descend into a quarter-squat, and jump again.

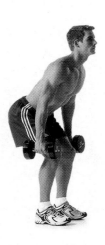 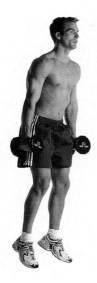

REVERSE HYPEREXTENSION

● Lie facedown, with your torso on a bench from the navel up, and your legs hanging off behind so they nearly touch the floor.

● Holding on to the sides of the bench, use your gluteals and hamstrings to lift your legs straight up into the air until they're just above parallel to the floor and your body forms a straight line. Hold that position for a few seconds, then return to the starting position.

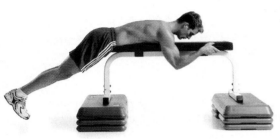

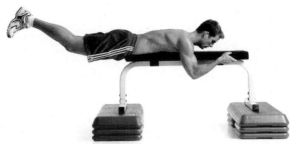

CABLE SINGLE-ARM EXTERNAL ROTATION

● Attach a stirrup handle to the low pulley. Grab the handle with your nondominant hand, and stand facing the weight stack, about a foot away. Lift your working arm into the finishing position of an upright row: upper arm parallel to the floor and forearm pointing straight down.

● Without allowing your upper arm to move up or down, rotate it so your forearm points toward the ceiling. Pause, then return to the starting position. Finish your set with that arm, then repeat with your other arm.

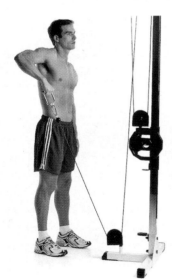

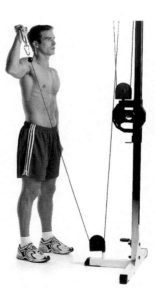

This workout series is adapted from *The Men's Health Home Workout Bible,* by Lou Schuler, with exercise programs by Michael Mejia, M.S., C.S.C.S., © 2002 by Rodale Inc. Available wherever books are sold.

Training Tips

HOW LOW CAN YOU GO?

Q **When I do squats, I can't go nearly as low as your models in *Men's Health* without my heels lifting off the floor. What am I doing wrong?**

D.M., NEW MILFORD, CONNECTICUT

A Squatting is a lot like being married: Some guys are good at it right away, but the rest of us need time, practice, and flexibility. When *Men's Health*'s own Muscle Guy, Lou Schuler, was a neophyte lifter, some guys convinced him he wouldn't get anything out of his squats unless he put his butt on his calves. So he tried it—and didn't go near a squat rack for the next 15 years.

This drill helped him get the motion right: Stand in front of a chair, and practice sitting back onto it. Notice how your heels never come off the floor? That's because you're shifting your center of gravity backward, leading with your butt, rather than starting the exercise with your knees moving forward.

How low you go is a function of hip-joint flexibility, and that's something you develop slowly, like your tolerance for your mother-in-law. Keep trying; you'll get better. Remember: A good marriage keeps you on your toes, but a good squat leaves you flat-footed.

BUCKLE UP?

Q **To be on the safe side, should I wear a weight belt when I lift?**

G.E., OAKLAND, CALIFORNIA

A For maximum deadlifts and squats, yes. For curls, no. A study in the *Journal of Strength and Conditioning Research* found that 44 percent of the male lifters at a typical health club used belts, and a third of those men wore them for every exercise. One guy even wore his when doing cardio. Our advice: Belt up when you're going for a personal record, but for everything else, let your back learn to brace itself.

TIMING IS EVERYTHING

Q **Some routines tell me how fast to lift the weights. Why does it matter?**

T.B., ANN ARBOR, MICHIGAN

A Your muscles have different jobs that need to be performed at different speeds. Researchers studying sprint kayakers had half of them train with fast repetitions. The other group took about 2 seconds to lift each weight. The ones who lifted slowly had better starts in kayak sprints, but the fast lifters had stronger finishes. So, different lifting speeds create different performance benefits. Slow down or speed up, and your muscles will respond accordingly.

Q **Should I use a "false grip" for the bench press?**

R.D., SAN DIEGO, CALIFORNIA

A Every time we see a guy using a false grip—thumbs under the bar instead of around it—we wonder why. We've heard it takes the forearms out of the lift, but that doesn't make sense. We think you should use your forearms more, not less. The top powerlifters believe that grip strength increases bench-press strength, and the more you can lift, the more muscle you can build. So put us down for "grab the bar and throttle it."

Second, the false grip is a wrist injury waiting to happen. It forces your wrists backward, into a hyperextended position, says Ken Kinakin, a chiropractor in Toronto and author of *Optimal Muscle Training* (optimalmuscletraining .com). Give it enough time, and you'll end up with bad wrists. Even worse, using a false grip increases the chance that you'll drop the bar on yourself. Out of the 20 deaths linked to weight training from 1999 to 2002, 12 were associated with bench presses, according to Pat Lombardi, Ph.D., an exercise researcher at the University of Oregon. You can't go back in

time and ask those guys if they were using a false grip, but deaths are deaths. Do you really want to go out with a barbell on your trachea and 15 guys asking how many more sets you have left?

Over-the-Counter Muscle

Researchers at Iowa State University recently reviewed nearly 250 vitamins, minerals, and sports supplements, and found that creatine and HMB are the only supplements that build both muscle mass and strength. Creatine tricks the body into delivering extra protein to the muscles, giving them more of the amino acids they need to grow. HMB (beta-hydroxy-beta-methylbutyrate) is thought to prevent breakdown of muscle tissue during strenuous exercise. Added to a strength-training program, HMB and creatine increase muscle growth by 200 percent more than strength training alone, says Steven Nissen, Ph.D., the lead study author. For best results, take each supplement twice a day.

Be More Eccentric

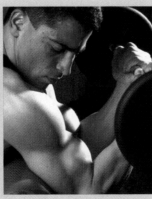

Lowering weights makes you stronger than lifting them. In a recent University of Texas study, researchers found that individuals who weight-trained using 75 percent eccentric (lowering) movements and 25 percent concentric (lifting) movements regained strength faster than those who spent more time on the concentric phase. One researcher speculates that eccentric movements do more to stimulate the muscle rebuilding process. Try curling a preacher-curl bar with two hands and lowering it with one.

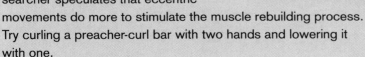

I hear there's a new testosterone tablet that dissolves under the gums. Will this help me build muscle?

J.O., LANSING, MICHIGAN

Don't do it, advises John R. White, Jr., P.A.-C., Pharm.D., professor of pharmacotherapy at Washington State University. It's extremely dangerous to mess with this hormone. You're asking

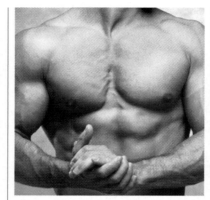

about Striant, prescribed for low levels of testosterone (as measured by a blood test). But for men with normal testosterone levels, the side effects include breast development, baldness, acne, anxiety, depression, and a huge increase in the risk of several cancers. Want to bulk up? Only work can take you there.

What are the most important numbers to keep track of in the gym?

A.C., HOUSTON

Expand Your Workout

You need to target your large muscle groups to build strength, power, and size, but don't neglect your "expansive muscles"—those thin, sheetlike muscles that cover the greatest surface area. Your expansive muscles (such as your trapezius and lats) have great potential for strength increases because they encompass such large areas of the body, says Alan Mikesky, Ph.D., director of the Human Performance and Biomechanics Laboratory at Indiana University-Purdue University at Indianapolis. Plus, by building these muscles using the guide that follows, they'll provide better support for smaller muscles as well as those with more mass.

EXPANSIVE MUSCLE	WHERE IT EXTENDS	HOW TO WORK IT
Trapezius	From the base of the neck to the middle of the back.	Shoulder shrugs, rows, pullups
Latissimus dorsi	From the lower back to the middle of the spine. It wraps around your sides and up to the upper arms.	Pullups, lat pulldowns, dumbbell pullovers, rows
Pectoralis major	From the collarbone down to the middle of the rib cage, or sternum. The narrow end of its fan shape extends out to the upper arm.	Chest presses, dips, pushups, dumbbell flies
Vastus lateralis	From the upper thighbone down to the kneecap.	Squats, leg presses, lunges, leg extensions
External oblique	From the ribs down to the iliac bone, a curved bone on your hips.	Lateral bridges, Russian twists, side bends

A Here's what you need to know to grow huge: (1) the number of repetitions you do, and (2) the amount of weight you lift. It's that simple. "The determinant of success is lifting more—either load or repetitions—in each successive workout," says Ian King, C.S.C.S., coauthor of *The Book of Muscle*. So if you're looking for bigger anything, ramp up at least one set of at least one exercise every time you hit the gym. As long as you do, you'll make progress. Tracking these two numbers will also tell you if you're resting enough between workouts. If you can't bump up either number, you need more time between workouts, or you need to decrease the number of sets you do in a given workout. If neither

of these changes results in muscle magic, you're simply putting your muscles under the same stress too often, says King. First, try subtle variations: Shift your grip, foot position, or sequence of exercises. Still not getting results? You're probably overtraining. Take time to rest (a couple of days, at least), then return with a new plan.

NEED A LIFT

Q **If I lift weights at lunch, I'm wiped out and sore for the rest of the day. How can I recover faster?**
C.P., BAY RIDGE, NEW YORK

A We're guessing you're working out too fast, so your mus-

cles don't have enough time to recover. Give yourself at least 90 seconds between exercises. Also, try reducing the weight you're lifting by 10 percent. Eat beforehand and drink a sports drink afterward to replace lost nutrients.

WAIT IT OUT

What a Difference a Day Makes

Walk, don't run, to the weight room. Canadian researchers have determined that you need to wait 24 hours after a bout of cardio in order to get the most out of lower-body strength training. In the study, men who cycled to fatigue, then waited 4 hours before their lower-body workouts, completed 25 percent fewer repetitions than those who did nothing before lifting. "But the day after, fatigue dissipated, and the number of repetitions was the same as with no aerobic training," says David Docherty, Ph.D., a professor of exercise science at the University of Victoria in Canada. Run or cycle on days when you do upper-body exercises.

LOOK INTO THE FUTURE

Delta Force

Researchers at Stanford University have discovered the protein that helps some muscles heal faster. Called Delta, this protein not only speeds the cell division necessary 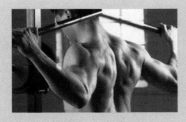 for muscles to repair themselves, but also keeps the division constant. The researchers envision a topical "Delta cream" that could potentially help decrease muscle recovery time, thereby speeding up the muscle-building process.

PICK A PART

You know you do it. When you check out a woman, you look at, um, certain parts. Hey, they stand out. We understand. And yet, you're really pursuing the whole woman in all of her glory. Not just a certain part.

Same goes for our own bodies. Sure we want to have a great all-around physique. Arms we're proud to wrap around our woman, a chest we're not afraid to bare in the bedroom, abs she can wash her clothes on. But the truth is, we focus on certain parts of our own bodies as well. Those abs, for example. Which is why the cover of *Men's Health* almost always shows a guy with great abs. We know what you're after. We read your mail.

This section satisfies the needs of those who have a favorite muscle—the one you like to work until you achieve perfection. No matter which part it is—your arms, abs, chest, shoulders, back, whatever—we'll help you achieve what you're looking for.

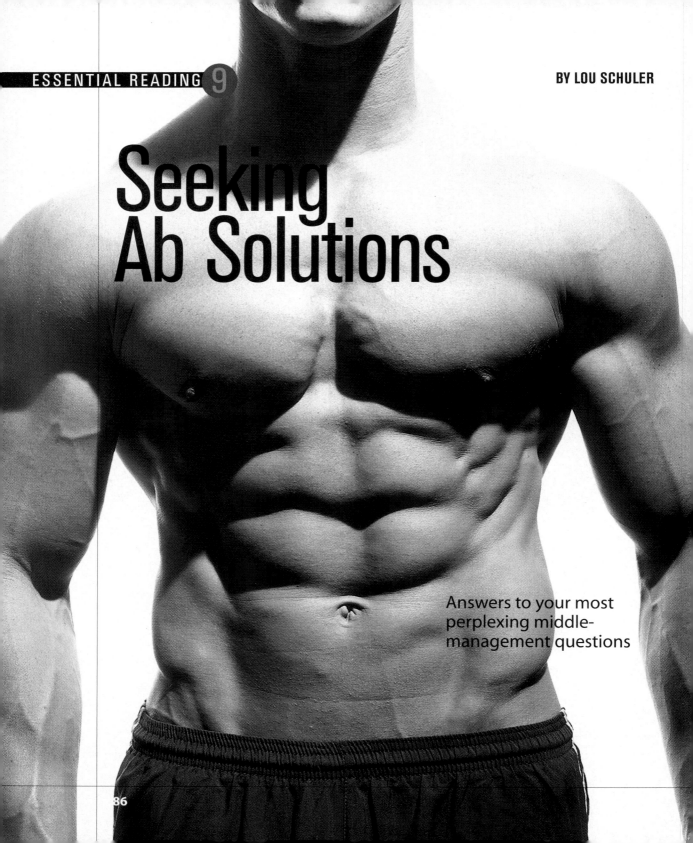

BY LOU SCHULER

Seeking Ab Solutions

Answers to your most perplexing middle-management questions

Every 36 minutes, a visitor to menshealth.com clicks on "Ask the Muscle Guy" and throws a question my way. Every 36 days, I answer one in my little corner of the *Malegrams* section of *Men's Health*. You ask 14,600 questions a year. I answer 10, one for each issue of the magazine. The ratio for questions related to abdominals is even worse. Out of perhaps 4,000, I answer maybe one a year in my column.

We decided the disparity between your need to know and my ability to tell is an abomination, and it's time we did something about it. On the following pages, I'll attach some A's to nine popular ab-related Q's. I can't answer all 4,000, but, on the plus side, I'm now 800 percent ahead of last year's pace.

Q: I'm very lean—less than 10 percent body fat—but I still have only two visible segments of my six-pack. How do I get the final four?

A: When I first started working out in a commercial gym, circa 1980, there was this guy who'd come in and start his workout with a set of full situps on a slant board, which was the opposite of what everyone else in that little proto-Bally's was doing back then. We were doing hundreds of cute little crunches while he was doing dozens of nasty situps. Guess who had the abs?

I like the full-range-of-motion ab exercises, as opposed to the truncated crunch variations, for three reasons: One, full situps

are harder, and I think harder is better. Two, they force other muscles in your thighs and trunk to help with the exercise, and I believe the more muscle you use, the more muscle you build. Nature didn't design your muscles to work in isolation; why try to build them that way? Three, their reputation as being hard on a healthy back is exaggerated. (There's some risk, but not more than in exercises such as reverse crunches, which no one regards as dangerous.)

Here's how to do the full situp on a slant board: Hook your feet under the braces, lower yourself until your lower back is flat against the bench, then pull yourself up to a full sitting position.

As you get better at it, you can lower the angle of the slant board and increase your knee angle—that is, put your butt farther from your heels. I like to do this exercise with straight legs. From that elongated position, first push your lower back against the board, flattening your spine, then start curling up.

Q: What's the best ab exercise?

A: Studies have shown that one exercise or another works certain abdominal muscles harder than other ab exercises do. But within each study, you'll find lots of variation from one participant to the next—what works the upper abs hardest for one person in the study might work the lower abs hardest for another. The best exercise for you is probably the one that feels as if it's working your muscles the most while you're doing it.

Examples: A couple of years ago, I started doing stability exercises for the first time. The best known of these is the plank, also

called the bridge, also called that damned painful thing you do on your elbows and toes. If you're a loyal *MH* reader, you've seen it a bunch of times—you rest your weight on your forearms and toes, pull your abs in tight, and hold your body in a straight line from shoulders to heels. After a few weeks of doing this twice a week—along with the similar side bridge, in which you rest your weight on one forearm and the outer edge of the same-side foot while holding your body straight as a pencil—I noticed muscles on the sides of my waist that I'd never seen before. I could feel those muscles working hard, and sure enough, those muscles grew.

Another time, mostly out of boredom, I decided to do sets of 100 crunches on a Swiss ball. My abs felt as if they'd been stoned (in the biblical sense), and within a couple of weeks, they looked distinctly more rocky.

Q: I've followed every bit of advice you've ever offered, and still have excess flesh right below my belly button. How do I get rid of it?

A: Since my advice hasn't worked, I went to a higher authority. "It's 100 percent diet, and it's the obvious stuff," says Jose Antonio, Ph.D., an adjunct professor of exercise sci-

ence at Florida Atlantic University. "Eliminate processed carbohydrates. If it comes in a package, don't eat it."

If you've already tried eliminating junk carbs—fiberless cereals, sodas, "low-fat" baked goods—try something more advanced: Separate carbohydrates and fat, so you never eat both in the same meal. Ideally, you alternate between the nonfat and the noncarb meals throughout the day, with each meal containing some protein. This is a technique recommended by John Berardi, C.S.C.S., a nutrition researcher at the University of Western Ontario who does individualized diet consultation at johnberardi.com.

It's easier to recommend than to implement. But I use it when I need to take off a pound or two of fat, and it works every time. A few examples of how to do it:

	NO FAT	NO (OR LOW) CARBS
Breakfast	High-fiber cereal with blueberries and nonfat milk	Eggs with low-fat meat
Lunch	Sandwich made with turkey breast, whole wheat bread, lettuce, tomatoes, and mustard	Tuna salad with mayonnaise
Dinner	Baked skinless chicken breast, sweet potato, and salad with nonfat dressing	Sirloin steak and mixed-green salad (which has very few carbohydrates) with olive oil–based dressing
Snack	Nonfat yogurt, fruit	Peanut butter

Q: My abs don't line up evenly. Is there anything I can do to make them straight?

A: Other than take away their show-tune collections, no, there's nothing you can do to straighten your abs. But look on the bright side: Even asymmetrical abs are still abs. And let's not forget that Owen McKibbin, the most popular cover model in *Men's Health* history, has crooked midbody muscles. (His ears are kind of funny looking, too.)

Q: How often should I work my abs?

A: I put this question to Ian King, C.S.C.S., an Australian strength coach and my coauthor on *The Book of Muscle*. "You can do ab exercises for injury prevention every day if you want," King says. But if you're looking to improve performance—that is, if you're trying to make your ab muscles bigger, stronger, or more powerful—you should leave at least a day between abdominal workouts.

The situp I talked about in the first question qualifies as a performance move. For injury prevention, King's favorite exercise is the "thin tummy," which strengthens the deep abdominal muscles that act like a corset to stabilize your hips and lower back. (The bridge and side bridge that I described in the second question fall into this category, too.)

Lie on your back on the floor, knees bent, feet flat. Place your hands over your midsection, so your thumbs touch your upper abs and your fingers spread across your lower abs. Now pull your abdominals in, so you can feel the increased tension just beneath your skin. Hold for 5 to 10 seconds while continuing to breathe (breathing makes the muscle contrac-

PEAK
performance

Well Centered
As you lose weight, crunches become less effective. (You're lifting less weight.) So add a medicine ball to your ab regimen to keep the ripples coming.

tion feel more intense), then release. Repeat for a total of 5 to 15 repetitions. That's one set, and plenty to start with. You can add one or two more sets when this seems easy.

Q: How do I get a torso like Brad Pitt's?

A: Find a mad scientist (try guyswholaughmaniacally.org, if you don't know any personally), have him build a time machine, go back to the spring of 1963, and arrange to be conceived by Mr. and Mrs. Pitt. Then simply follow Brad's diet and workout routine for the next 39 years, and you'll have abs just like his. I guarantee this program will work—in fact, it's never failed to produce Brad Pitts.

Q: How much aerobic exercise should I do if I want my abs to show?

A: I can't think of a reason you have to do any. If you go on the theory that visible abs are a combination of (a) well-developed abdominal muscles and (b) very little body fat hiding them, then the two most important concerns for you should be . . .

1. exercise that builds visible muscle, and

2. a combination of diet and exercise that creates a calorie deficit, forcing your body to burn excess fat

On point number one, endurance exercise is clearly pointless. No amount of jogging is going to help build your abdominal muscles. And on point two, you choose aerobic exercise only if you decide that you can't possibly create that calorie deficit through strength training and a disciplined diet.

Some men are predisposed to be good at endurance exercise and not good at building muscle mass. These guys, if no one else, should find it easier to lose their excess belly fat through aerobics.

As for me, I've never been able to run farther than 5 miles at a time (and that was back when I was trying), so using endurance exercise for fat loss was never a very effective option.

A lot of guys try to do high volumes of both types of exercise, figuring that if you burn twice as many calories, you get your abs in half the time. I think this strategy is fine if you're 16 and your parents give you a nice allowance. But let's say you're an adult with a job and other sources of stress. ("Dad,

Test Your Ab-Q

True or False: Crunches on a Swiss ball are better than crunches on the floor.

True. A 2000 study at the University of Waterloo in On-

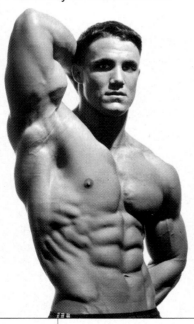

tario compared crunches on the floor with those on a ball and found that the rectus abdominis, the six-pack muscle, worked more than twice as hard on the ball. (The obliques worked four times harder.) The real discovery here is that the basic crunch is a pretty weak exercise, forcing the rectus abdominis to work at just 21 percent of its maximum effort.

True or False: It's best to do ab exercises in the morning, when your body is fresh.

False. Your spinal disks fill with fluid overnight, which makes them much more prone to injury in the morning than later in the day, when they've had a chance to return to normal hydration levels. All ab

exercises involve bending the spine, a movement that challenges its disks even under the best conditions. Stick to sex in the morning, and work your abs some other time.

True or False: A situp with straight legs is more dangerous to your lower back than one with bent legs.

False. The straight-leg situp has long had a bad-back rep, based on the idea that it forces the hip-flexor muscles to contract so hard that they damage the soft tissues in your lower back. But a Swedish study published in 1997 found that the hip flexors work 111 percent harder during the bent-knee situp. Make no mistake: Straight is great.

why is Mommy crying so hard? It was just an old picture—I can draw sunflowers better than that guy!")

You have to figure out how much exercise you can recover from, not how much you can do. If your body can't recover from the extra exercise you do in the pool or on the road, it makes no sense to do it.

Q: I need a new ab exercise. Do you have any killers?

A: I think this one's called supine spinal flexion with inappropriately aggressive arm actions. I shorten that to "ass-kicker."

Lie on your back on the floor, knees bent and feet flat. Hold your fists up by your cheeks. Sit up, and, as you do, throw a punch or a combination of punches.

It's most intense when you stop short of a full situp position and throw the punches from there. You'll feel action from abdominal muscles you never knew you had.

You can make it more satisfyingly aggressive by having a training partner stand and hold a pillow or punching bag over your hips, so you actually can hit something with your punches.

Q: What's best for abs—high reps, low reps, or something in between?

A: All of the above. High reps will challenge the smaller, more endurance-oriented muscle fibers. Low reps with heavy resistance will hit the fibers that produce strength and power. And at least a couple of times a week, do isometric holds of 30 to 60 seconds on the bridges and other injury-prevention exercises.

BY ALWYN COSGROVE, C.S.C.S.

Arm Yourself

For bigger guns, take aim with these biceps-building moves

Here's a two-part quiz. Question one: Are you happy with the size of your biceps? Question two: Why not? Okay, loaded questions. The only way you answer yes to number one is if you're female or a yoga instructor.

All men want big biceps. Trouble is, most guys have been doing the same two or three arm exercises since the ninth grade, when they first learned to curl a dumbbell. If you adopted that status quo philosophy in other areas of your life, you'd still be buying

Poison cassettes, playing Atari, and rolling up the cuffs of your jeans. Times change. So should your workout.

Using variations of the basic curl, I'll show you how to graduate to a higher level of arm training. You'll combine curl exercises that you've never seen with lifting techniques that you've never tried, for a biceps workout guaranteed to add inches. Plus, you'll learn how to curl for maximum strength, explosive power, and even fat loss—all of which lead back to your ultimate goal of thicker, more defined arms.

Class is starting. Now cut that mullet, and get to work.

Curls for Muscle

Your biceps muscles are composed of both fast-twitch and slow-twitch fibers. So the key to maximizing arm size is to make sure you work all of these fibers. Try this three-move routine twice a week for 4 weeks. It hits your fast-twitch fibers with heavy weights and low repetitions, a combination of your fast- and slow-twitch fibers with medium weights and repetitions, and your slow-twitch fibers with light weights and high repetitions. You'll perform the first exercise with your arms behind your body, the second with your arms in line with your body, and the third with your arms in front of your body, to help hit the entire complex of muscles that make up your biceps. Do the workout as a triset, performing one set of each of the three exercises, with no rest in between, before beginning your second set of each move. Complete a total of three trisets.

DUMBBELL INCLINE CURL (6 reps) Set an incline bench to a 45-degree angle. (More upright is easier; flatter is harder, but potentially tougher on your shoulders.) Grab a pair of dumbbells, and lie on your back on the bench. Let your arms hang straight down from your shoulders, and turn your palms forward.

Without allowing your upper arms to move forward, slowly curl the weights up as high as you can. Then, without pausing, take 5 seconds to lower the dumbbells back to the starting position.

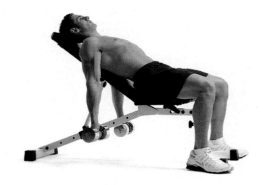

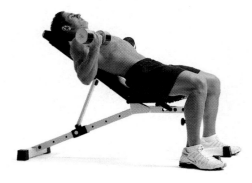

DUMBBELL OFFSET CURL (12 reps) Grab a pair of dumbbells with an offset, underhand grip, so that your little finger is pressed against the inside head of the dumbbell and your palms are facing forward. Sit at the end of a bench, and hold the dumbbells at arm's length at your sides.

Without allowing your upper arms to move forward, take 2 seconds to curl the weights up as high as you can. Pause for 1 second, then take 3 seconds to lower the dumbbells back to the starting position.

bench. Let your arms hang straight down from your shoulders, and turn your palms to face each other.

Without allowing your upper arms to move backward, slowly curl the weights up as high as you can. Pause for 1 second, then take 1 second to lower the dumbbells back to the starting position.

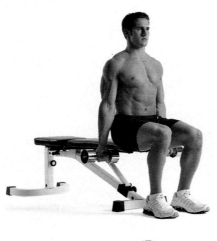

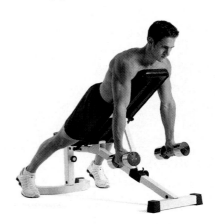

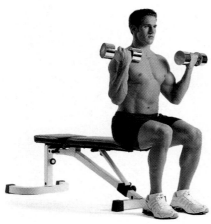

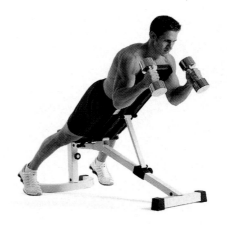

DECLINE HAMMER CURL (25 reps) Set an incline bench to a 45-degree angle. (More upright is easier; flatter is harder.) Grab a pair of dumbbells, and lie chest-down on the

Curls for Fat Loss

Who would use curls for fat loss? You would, if you wanted to increase your energy expenditure and work your arms without spending more time at the gym. After all, your gut shouldn't be the only beneficiary of your fat-fighting workout. Add curls to virtually any lower-body dumbbell exercise—lunges, step-ups, squats—and beef up your biceps while you burn off the pounds. Go one step further and incorporate an overhead press after you curl, and you'll target your shoulders and triceps, too. Here's one of my favorite curl combos. Do three sets.

DUMBBELL LUNGE, CURL, AND PRESS (8 to 10 reps) Grab a pair of dumbbells, and hold them at your sides. Stand with your feet hip-width apart.

Step forward with your left leg, and lower your body down and forward until you can touch the dumbbells to the floor next to your left foot. Your left lower leg should be perpendicular to the floor.

In one move, curl the weights to shoulder level as you push yourself quickly back to a standing position. Then press the dumbbells above your head until your arms are almost straight (not shown). Lower the weights to the starting position and repeat, stepping forward with your right leg this time. That's one repetition.

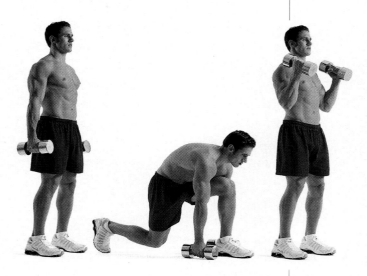

Arms Deal

How to buy big guns

For some men, getting bigger biceps is as easy as dozing off. That's because they put their twigs under the knife and wake up with biceps implants.

During the 90-minute procedure, a 1½-inch incision is made under the armpit, and a solid silicone implant is fitted into the biceps muscle. "The implants are very soft, so when the muscle flexes, the implant moves right with it," says J. Howell Tiller, M.D., a Miami-based plastic surgeon, "although the biggest complaint I get is from people wishing they were softer."

Patients wake up with soreness and must elevate their arms for a couple of days. Tiller says people can use their arms immediately, but they should avoid arm exercises for 4 to 6 weeks. There are cosmetic risks, like asymmetry, and the medical risks of any surgery—infection, bleeding, scarring, nerve damage, and anesthesia problems. Plus they're a bitch to resell on eBay.

Implants cost $7,000. For another grand, you can have triceps work, too. (Of course, you can get a personal trainer and a deluxe home gym for much less.) Visit implants.com for more information.

Curls for Strength

There's a simple link between strength and muscle: Get stronger, and you'll be able to lift heavier weights; lift heavier weights, and you'll build more muscle. You gain strength fastest by shoring up your weaknesses, and the number-one strength-limiting factor for most men is their grip. (Think of your arm as a chain. The weakest link is your forearm, which provides grip strength. Strengthen your forearm, and you allow the stronger part of the chain—your biceps—to work longer and harder.) Use the moves below to add more iron to your arm workout and more muscle to your arms. The exercises utilize towels to create oversize grips, which force your forearms to work harder than usual. Try the workout below twice a week for 3 weeks. When you switch back to your normal grip, you'll find you're stronger than ever. Do three to five sets of the first exercise, then three to five sets of the second exercise. Rest 90 seconds after each set.

FAT-GRIP BARBELL CURL (4 to 6 reps)

Wrap two hand towels around a barbell, and grab the towel-wrapped bar with an underhand, shoulder-width grip. Hold the bar at arm's length in front of your thighs.

Without moving your upper arms forward or changing your posture, slowly curl the bar as high as you can. Then, without pausing, take 3 seconds to lower it back to the starting position.

DUMBBELL TOWEL CURL (4 to 6 reps)

Loop a hand towel around each handle of a pair of dumbbells, and hold the weights by grasping the ends of each towel. Hold the dumbbells at arm's length next to the sides of your legs, your palms facing each other.

Without moving your upper arms, slowly curl the dumbbells as high as you can. Then, without pausing, take 3 seconds to lower them back to the starting position.

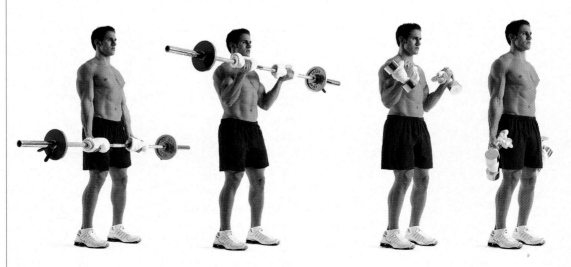

Curls for Power

If you're like most guys in the gym, you're familiar with the "cheat" curl—just not this version. That's because men like to curl as much weight as they can, even if they can't do it with good form. So they end up swaying their upper body back and forth, like one of those dunking-bird pendulums you find in novelty shops. Not only does it look stupid, but it's a good way to throw out your back, as well. There is a benefit to lifting fast and extra-heavy, though, if you do it right. By focusing on speed and strength at the same time, you'll work your deepest, largest muscle fibers, a process that helps create thicker, denser-looking muscles. (Think NFL linebacker.) Use the power cheat curl to get the benefits of heavy, explosive arm curls, without the danger to your lower back. Do four or five sets.

DUMBBELL POWER CHEAT CURL (2 or 3 reps) Grab a pair of heavy dumbbells, and hold them at arm's length next to your sides, your palms facing each other. Lean forward at your hips, and bend your legs until the dumbbells are next to and in line with your knees, or just above them.

Curl the dumbbells, push your hips forward, and straighten your legs all at the same time, until you're standing upright and the dumbbells are almost resting on your shoulders. Lower the dumbbells back to the starting position, and repeat.

Sore Subject

When I work out, all my muscles get sore from time to time, except my biceps. What am I doing wrong?

E.B., KITCHENER, ONTARIO

We're professionally obligated to point out that muscle soreness has no proven correlation to gains in size or strength. But, as muscleheads ourselves, we know exactly what you mean. We trust soreness. It's like anger—a proof-of-passion seal that only you can appreciate.

Try heavy negative chinups. Strap on a dip belt (a lifting belt with a chain or rope that holds additional weight), load it with something heavy, climb up the chinning bar so you're in the finishing position of a chinup (underhand grip), and then slowly lower yourself. Try to last 30 seconds. The next day, you'll feel the passion.

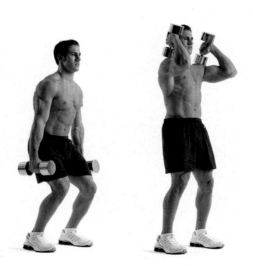

Shoulders Above

Two easy exercises that will round out your shoulders

To build shoulders as big as small planets, you need to train the whole shoulder. But unless you live in cell block B, you don't have time to do separate exercises for your front, side, and rear deltoids, as well as your rotator cuffs. So try these two total-shoulder moves from James Cavin, C.S.C.S., a Massachusetts trainer. Do one set of each exercise with one arm, then switch arms. Do three sets of 12 repetitions on each side.

HIGH-PULLEY CROSSOVER Stand with your right side next to the high pulley, and hold the handle in your left hand at head level on the right side of your body.

Pull your left arm down and back while rotating your palm, so that it's facing behind you. Finish with your arm at an angle below your shoulder and on the left side of your body.

LOW-PULLEY CROSSOVER Stand with your right side next to the low pulley, and hold the handle in your left hand, next to your right hip—as if you were about to unsheath a sword.

Pull your left arm up and out in front of your body while rotating your palm up. Finish with your hand at an angle above your shoulder on the left side of your body.

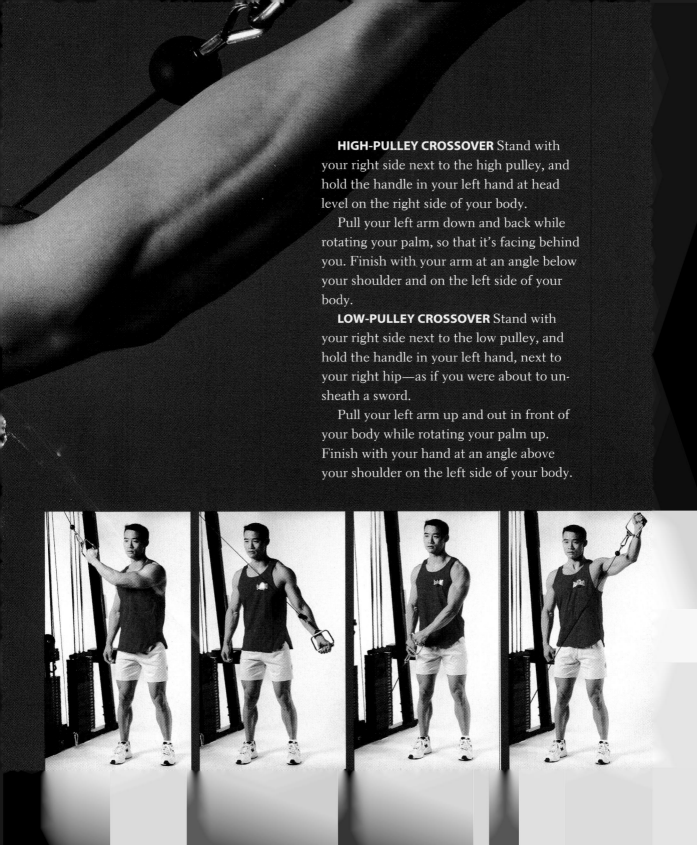

A Bolder Shoulder

If you want your shoulders to have great definition in the back as well as the front, you need to hit the rear head of the deltoid. To achieve that, do the following exercises as a superset—do one after the other, with no rest in between. Knock out two or three sets of 8 to 12 repetitions, resting 15 seconds after each set, suggests Alwyn Cosgrove, C.S.C.S., owner of Results Fitness in Santa Clarita, California.

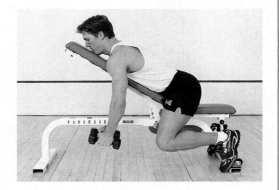

45-Degree Dumbell Raise (shown)

Lie facedown on an incline bench with a 5- to 8-pound dumbbell in each hand.

Holding the dumbbells with your thumbs pointing up, lift the weights up and outward at a 45-degree angle.

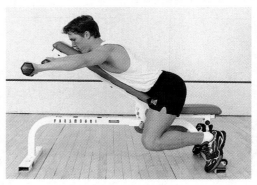

The second exercise is a cable row with rope. Using a rope attachment, sit at a cable-row station. Keeping your back straight, pull the rope up toward your neck rather than toward your chest. At the end of the movement (when the rope is at chin level), your upper arms should be parallel to the floor.

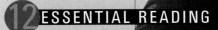

Build pecs you
can be proud of
with this killer workout

Go Bare-Chested

The average guy can bench-press 135 pounds. Poor guy. Follow our rules, and your chest will never be mistaken for his. The chest is a primary muscle group that requires other, secondary muscle groups—mainly the shoulders and triceps—to assist in every exercise. If you work your shoulders and triceps beforehand, they'll quit on you before your chest works hard enough to grow. The smartest order: chest first, shoulders second, triceps last.

The Payoff

Better sex. A stronger, bigger chest will fill out your shirt in such a way that women will be inspired to remove that shirt. In bed, the ever-popular missionary position gives her a satisfying view of your chest—and you'll be able to support yourself longer.

More power. Stronger chest muscles make it easier to push off opponents in any contact sport, whether your game is football, basketball, martial arts, or hockey.

A stronger swing. Forehand strokes in tennis and sidearm throws in baseball rely on powerful chest muscles for velocity, in addition to your core musculature.

A knockout punch. The chest's primary objective is to move the arms forward, so developing pectoral strength helps you deliver more energy into your target.

The Main Move

The barbell bench press is the granddaddy of all chest exercises, working more muscle fibers in the chest than any other move.

BARBELL BENCH PRESS Lie on a bench with your head, torso, and hips pressed against it and your feet spread wide and flat on the floor. Grab the bar with a full overhand grip (thumbs wrapped around the bar). Place your hands slightly wider than shoulder-width apart, remove the bar from the uprights, and hold it with straight arms over your collarbone.

Pull your shoulder blades together. Lower the bar, slowly and in control, until it touches your chest just below your nipples. Then press the weight up and slightly back, so it finishes above your collarbone again. You can lock your elbows or stop just short. Keep your shoulder blades pulled back.

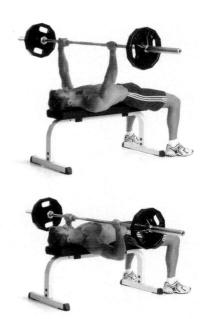

Mix and Max

Vary your grip. Your hand position helps determine how your chest develops. A wider grip emphasizes your chest, while a narrower grip involves more of your triceps and deltoids.

Change tools. You'll lift less weight with dumbbells, but since they allow your hands to move independently of each other, it will be easier to keep your hands directly in line with your elbows, reducing your risk of injury.

Adjust your approach. Instead of conforming to the standard three sets of three exercises that most men use to work their chest muscles, perform one set of seven different exercises. This approach conditions the muscles from seven specific angles, instead of three, in one workout, utilizing a higher percentage of muscle fibers for maximum overall growth.

Your Power Plan

To develop the best chest, you need to vary the ways your shoulders and triceps are involved. Your chest recruits extra support from your triceps near the top of the bench press; your deltoids assist mostly at the bottom; and both help your chest in the middle. These six exercises involve your secondary muscle groups to ensure a smooth movement throughout the bench press. After your bench-press routine, pick one exercise from each section: A (upper chest and deltoids), B (middle chest), and C (lower chest and triceps). Then build your program using the chart below. You'll get a custom-made workout that keeps your chest muscles guessing and growing. After a week of lifting, you'll start to see and feel the power.

DUMBBELL INCLINE PRESS (A) Lie on an incline bench with a dumbbell in each hand (palms forward), your arms extended straight above your chest.

The Right Workout for You

Build your perfect chest with this checklist.

YOUR LEVEL	WORK YOUR CHEST . . .	SETS OF EACH EXERCISE	REPETITIONS PER SET	SPEED OF EACH REP	REST BETWEEN SETS
Beginner	Three times a week	1–3	10–15	3–4 seconds up, 3–4 seconds down	30–60 seconds
Intermediate	Twice a week	2–4	6–12	1–3 seconds up, 1–3 seconds down	60–120 seconds
Advanced	Twice a week	3–5	3–6	1 second up, 1–2 seconds down	90–240 seconds

Lower the dumbbells until they're resting along the sides of your chest. Pause, then press the weights back up. (Hold them farther apart to target the front deltoids.)

Get more: Instead of keeping the bench fixed at one angle, try lowering it one notch from the highest angled position for your first set, then continue lowering the angle one notch after each set.

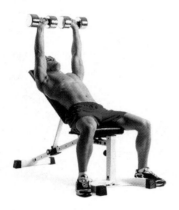

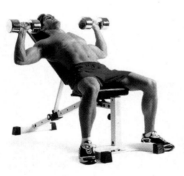

PARALLEL DIP (A) Grab the parallel bars of a dip station with a neutral grip, and lift yourself so your arms are straight but not locked. Bend your knees, and cross your ankles.

Slowly lower your body by bending your elbows until your upper arms are at least parallel to the floor. (The farther you lower

yourself, the harder your deltoids work to push you back up.) Pause, then push yourself back to the starting position, keeping your elbows unlocked at the top to maintain tension on your chest muscles.

Get more: If you're too strong to benefit from the specified number of repetitions, wear a dip belt (start with about 15 percent of your body weight). If you're not strong enough, take 2 seconds to lower yourself, step up to get into the starting position, and repeat.

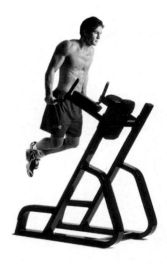

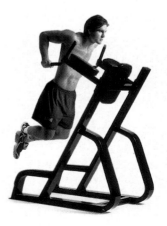

DUMBBELL FLY (B) Grab a pair of dumbbells that are lighter than those you use for bench presses. Lie on a bench, holding the dumbbells with a neutral grip (palms facing each other) above the middle of your pecs, arms straight up.

Maintaining a slight bend in your elbows, lower the dumbbells down and back until your upper arms are parallel to the floor and in line with your ears. Then use your chest to pull the weights back up to the starting position, following the same arclike route in reverse. Keep your shoulder blades pinched together throughout, and flex your pecs at the top of the movement.

Get more: Use an overhand grip to lower the dumbbells until your upper arms are parallel to the floor. As you use your chest to pull the weights back up, slowly rotate your palms so they face each other about halfway up and face toward you at the top of the move.

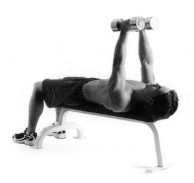

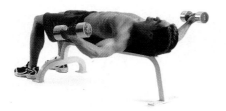

Challenging Changeups

Incline Bench Press

Lie on an incline bench set at a 15- to 30-degree angle, with your arms extended and the bar above your chin.

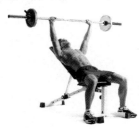

Lower the bar, moving it very subtly forward so that it finishes close to your collarbone. The angle of this lift places more of the emphasis on the upper (or clavicular) part of your chest.

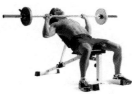

Plyometric Pushup

Assume the basic pushup position on a well-padded carpet or exercise mat. Lower yourself to the bottom position, then quickly push up with enough force so your hands come off the floor. Catch yourself with your elbows slightly bent, and go immediately into the next repetition.

Decline Bench Press

Lie on a decline bench set at a 30- to 45-degree angle, with your shins hooked beneath the leg supports.

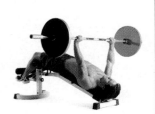

Lower the bar to an inch or two above your chest, pause, then press it back up. The angle of this lift targets the lower chest and decreases the range of motion, so you'll lift heavier weights than on a flat bench.

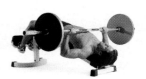

Swiss Ball Bench Press

Bench-press while lying on a Swiss ball so that your head, neck, and upper back are in contact with the ball. This teaches your proprioceptive fibers—the microscopic nerves responsible for keeping your body balanced at all times—to work more effectively with your chest muscles.

STANDING HIGH-CABLE CROSSOVER (B)

Attach two stirrup handles to the high cables of a cable-crossover station, and stand sideways to the weight stack. Grab the left handle with your left hand and the right handle with your right, and stand in the middle of the station. You may also want to take a step back; it's best to start with tension in the cables so there's resistance throughout the movement. Pull your shoulder blades back, and keep your elbows slightly bent.

Pull the handles down in a wide arc in front of your body until your hands just pass each other in front of your midsection. Pause, then return to the starting position.

Get more: Resist the urge to lean forward, because that prevents your chest from doing the work. You can reduce forward momentum and add weight by placing one foot slightly ahead of the other, while keeping them shoulder-width apart.

DUMBBELL DECLINE PRESS (C) Lie on a decline bench with your shins hooked beneath the leg supports. Grab a pair of dumbbells, and hold them above your head with your arms extended but not locked.

Lower the dumbbells to the outer edges of your chest, just below your nipples. Pause, then press them back up above your head.

Get more: A decline position shrinks your range of motion, making it easier to lift heavier weights. Start with dumbbells that are 15 to 20 percent heavier than you typically lift when lying flat.

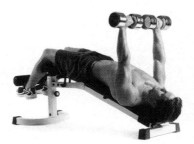

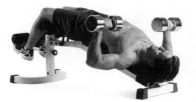

MEDICINE BALL PUSHUP (C) Kneel and place your hands along the sides of a medicine ball, spreading your fingers wide to help grip the surface (a soccer ball or basketball will also work). The space between your thumbs and index fingers should be diamond-shaped. Balance your weight on the ball, then slowly extend your legs behind you to assume the pushup position.

Lower your body until your chest touches your hands. Pause, then slowly press yourself back up to the starting position.

Get more: Perform one set to failure—the point at which you can't do any more repetitions. Then immediately move to your

knees, and continue until you reach failure again. Decreasing the load this way allows you to push your muscles beyond their usual state of fatigue.

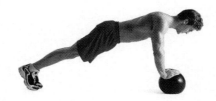

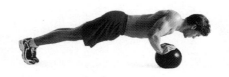

Meet Your Muscles

Your chest is composed of two muscle groups—the pectoralis major and the pectoralis minor

1. The pectoralis major, the larger layer and the one lying closer to the skin, is divided into three parts: the clavicular, which starts high at the collarbone; the abdominal, which originates at your external oblique muscles; and the sternocostal, which starts at the breastbone. Each stretches across your chest in a

fan shape, starting wide at the center of your body, then tapering at the side of your body to attach to the top of the humerus, the bone in your upper arm.

2. The pectoralis minor is a thinner, more triangular muscle that lies beneath the pectoralis major. It starts along the third, fourth, and fifth ribs and stretches to connect to the shoulder blade. It is largely used to pull up on the ribs

during heavy breathing. Together, the pectoralis major and pectoralis minor are responsible for rotating your upper arms and moving them across your body horizontally, as well as flexing the shoulder joints.

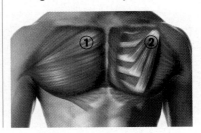

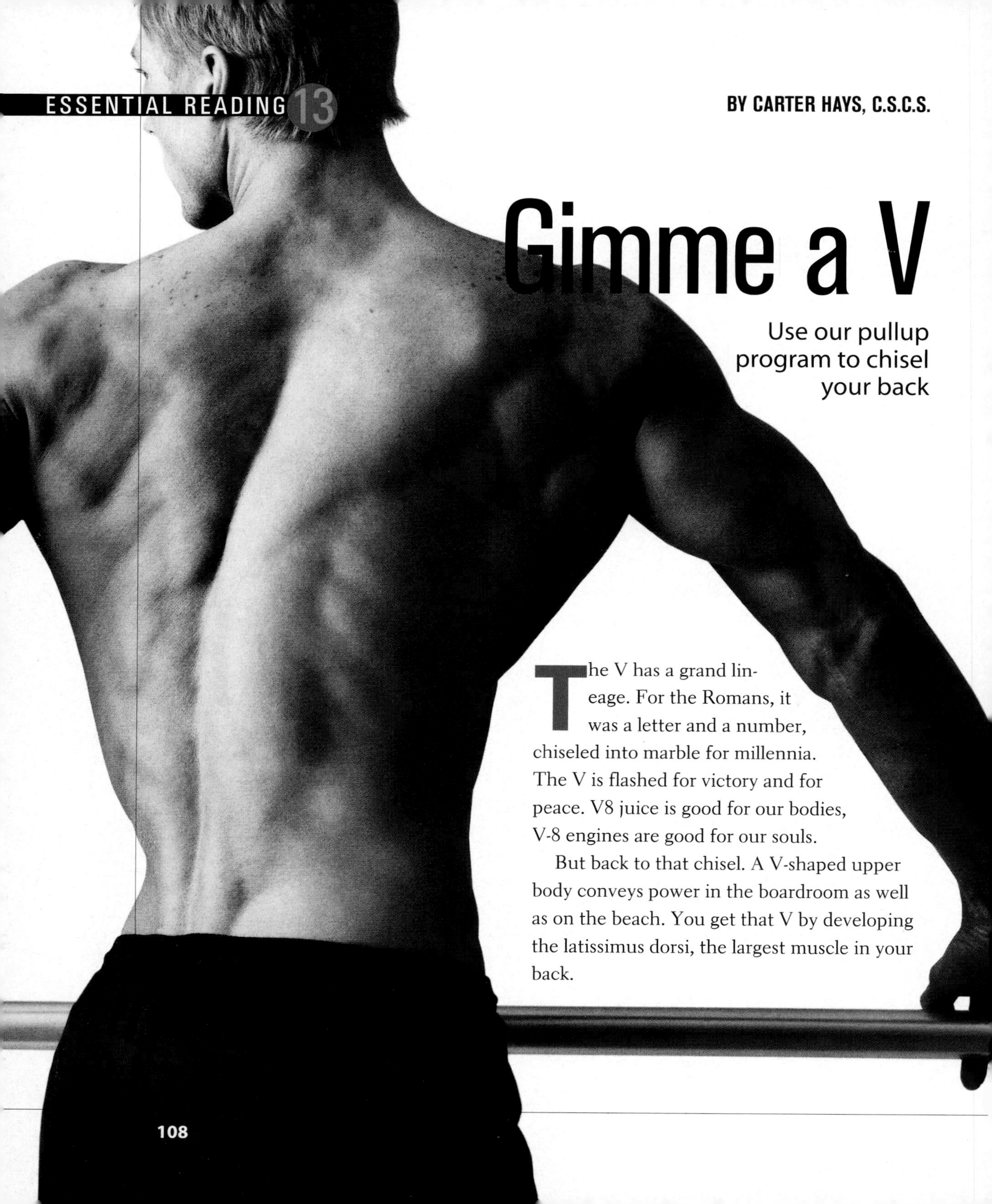

BY CARTER HAYS, C.S.C.S.

Gimme a V

Use our pullup
program to chisel
your back

The V has a grand lin-
eage. For the Romans, it
was a letter and a number,
chiseled into marble for millennia.
The V is flashed for victory and for
peace. V8 juice is good for our bodies,
V-8 engines are good for our souls.

But back to that chisel. A V-shaped upper
body conveys power in the boardroom as well
as on the beach. You get that V by developing
the latissimus dorsi, the largest muscle in your
back.

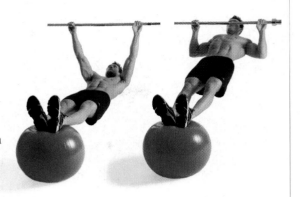

Pullups can deliver you to V-ness. They require strength, flexibility, and balance; they recruit muscles from your back, shoulders, arms, and core. Whether you call them pullups or chinups (see "What's the Diff?" below), they work.

Last year, I began training Mike, a man in his mid 40s who had never been able to do a pullup, and Zach, a 23-year-old who could easily do 15 repetitions but was dissatisfied with his back size. Each client used the following program, and each achieved his goal.

Get a Grip

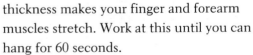

Unless you strengthen your grip, it will fail long before your arms, shoulders, or back.

STATIC HANG Grab the bar with an overhand grip, and hang with your arms straight. Once you can hang for 60 seconds, wrap a towel around the bar. The thickness makes your finger and forearm muscles stretch. Work at this until you can hang for 60 seconds.

Recruit Support

Your core connects your upper- and lower-body musculature. So improving core strength will keep your head, shoulders, hips, knees, and ankles properly aligned throughout the pullup.

SWISS BALL REVERSE PUSHUP On a Smith machine or squat rack, secure a bar

3 to 4 feet above the floor. Lie under the bar, and grab it with an overhand grip that's slightly wider than shoulder width. Hang at arm's length with your body in a straight line, and place your lower legs on a Swiss ball.

Keeping your body rigid, pull your chest to the bar. Pause, then lower yourself back to the starting position. Perform 12 repetitions.

What's the Diff?
Pullups and Chinups
Some trainers say a pullup uses an overhand grip (palms facing away from you), while a chinup is performed with an underhand grip. We at *Men's Health* go along with that, for clarity. Others say they're all chinups and that the overhand and neutral (palms facing each other) grips are variations. But "chinup" is misleading because you're supposed to lift your chin well past the bar, until your chest is even with the bar. Chinups work the biceps more and place less strain on your shoulders. Pullups require more forearm strength. Both work your back equally.

Boost Endurance

In a deadlift, the weight travels less than 1 foot. In a pullup, your body weight travels about 4 feet. That's tiring. You need to improve your muscular endurance.

GRAVITY GAMES Using a step (or a boost from a partner), hoist your chest to the bar. Then lower yourself slowly—try for a count of 12 before your arms are straight. Complete a set of six to eight repetitions.

Add Weight

As you become proficient at pullups, add weight to your frame to make the critical muscles work harder.

WEIGHTED PULLUP Add 10 percent of your body weight by attaching weight plates to a dip belt. (Or, if you can, hold a dumbbell between your feet.) Once you can do 12 pullups, increase the weight by 50 percent.

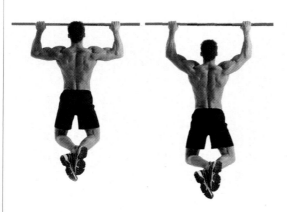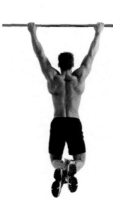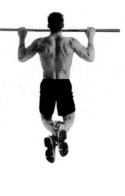

Break Your Own Record

A pullup champion tells you how

Former Marine Alan Sharkany, Jr., holds the world records for the most pullups in an hour (239) and the most in 24 hours (2,101). His advice has Zen-like simplicity, starting with this: "The key to growth is getting on the bar consistently." So get on it, maggot! And listen up:

Set flexible goals. Don't pressure yourself to perform a specific number of repetitions. This way, you'll eliminate failure and be more willing to get back up there.

Stop halfway. Never compromise form for repetitions. If you're partway up and can't reach the top without swinging your body, just hold yourself at the halfway point for 4 to 5 seconds.

Advance with caution. Pushing your muscles to fatigue too frequently doesn't let them recover and grow, so stop if you begin to feel pain. If you can't do four pullups, try to do a set of two, then rest and do another set of two. Then try to do a set of 1½. You'll boost your total without trying to do it all at once.

DROP-SET PULLUP After performing 12 weighted pullups, remove the weight and do as many unweighted pullups as you can. Working the muscles to failure makes them bigger, building your V. Do this only once every three workouts, or you risk over-training.

Forget Form

These variations challenge your muscles from unusual angles, spurring the growth that will complete your V.

STERNUM PULLUP Place your hands in an underhand grip. Pull your body up to the bar while leaning your torso back and bending your knees. Keep your back arched, and pull your head away from the bar. Touch your lower chest to the bar, so your body forms a 45-degree angle with the ground. Try to complete 12 repetitions.

HANGING-TOWEL PULLUP Place two hand towels over the bar at shoulder width. Grab both halves of each towel just below the bar.

Pull your chest to the bar. Your body travels a longer distance than in a standard pullup because you start lower. As this gets easier, start with your hands halfway down the towel. You won't be able to pull your chest to the bar, but the instability will force you to fight your body's tendency to swing. Aim for 12 reps.

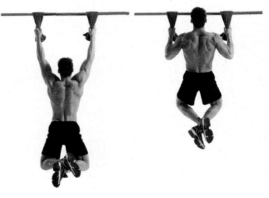

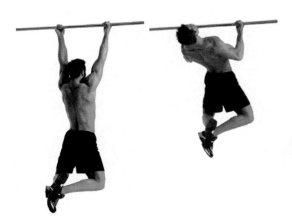

A Portable Bar

You've got a doorway, right? Then you can have a pullup bar. We looked at six home versions, and our favorite is the Door Gym. It requires no mounting hardware, is very sturdy, has comfortable grips, and gives you the options of neutral, underhand, and overhand grips. $40 from bodytrends.com

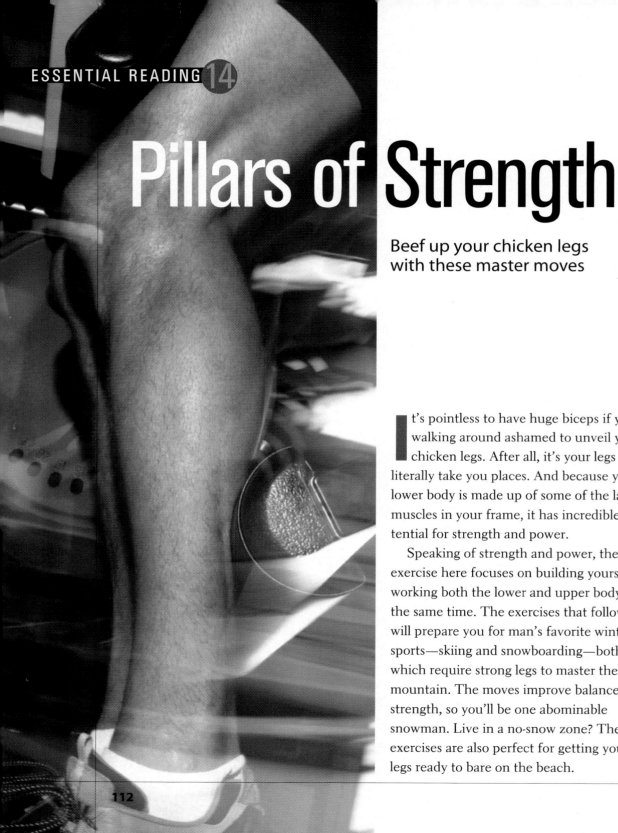

Pillars of Strength

Beef up your chicken legs
with these master moves

It's pointless to have huge biceps if you're walking around ashamed to unveil your chicken legs. After all, it's your legs that literally take you places. And because your lower body is made up of some of the largest muscles in your frame, it has incredible potential for strength and power.

Speaking of strength and power, the first exercise here focuses on building yours, working both the lower and upper body at the same time. The exercises that follow it will prepare you for man's favorite winter sports—skiing and snowboarding—both of which require strong legs to master the mountain. The moves improve balance and strength, so you'll be one abominable snowman. Live in a no-snow zone? These exercises are also perfect for getting your legs ready to bare on the beach.

A Powerful Combination

Build leg- and upper-body muscle with this eight-step exercise that works the whole body. Strength coach John Davies, author of *Renegade Training for Football,* calls this "The Bear," and it is. It's not for novices— and even experienced lifters may want to go through the moves with just a bar at first. If you can handle it, you'll boost your strength, size, and explosive power.

THE BEAR Hold the barbell in front of your thighs with a shoulder-width overhand grip, your knees slightly bent, your upper body bent forward slightly, and your back straight.

Dip your knees, shrug your shoulders, and, rising up on your toes, explosively pull the bar to chest level. "Catch" it on your front shoulders by dropping under it into a partial squat, as you turn your elbows underneath the bar so your palms face up. Your upper arms should be parallel to the floor when the bar lands on your shoulders.

Lower your body into a full front squat—

or at least until your thighs are parallel to the floor—by pushing your hips back and bending your knees as much as possible. Keep your back slightly arched in its natural alignment.

In one move, drive your feet into the floor, straighten your knees, and press the barbell over your head until your elbows lock.

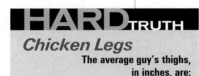

Pause, then lower the barbell behind your head and rest it on your upper back, as you would when performing a squat.

Lower your body into a full back squat— like the front squat, except for the position of the barbell.

In one move, drive your feet into the floor and straighten your knees as you press the barbell over your head.

Pause, then return the barbell to the starting position. That's one repetition.

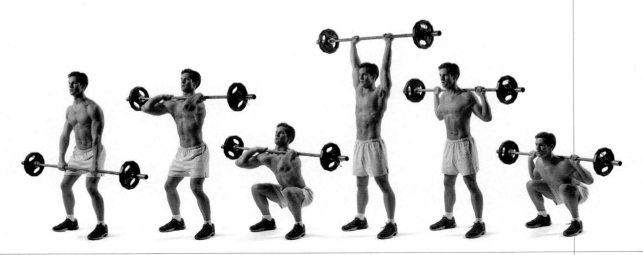

Get a Leg Up

Looking for the best one-stop leg exercise? Try the plate drag. It beats another session at the leg-curl machine in three ways: It challenges your back, abs, and hamstrings, says Tanya Miszko, Ed.D., C.S.C.S., a research exercise physiologist at the VA Medical Center in Atlanta. New beef will be popping out all over. Here's how to do it:

Plate Drag

Lie on your back with your legs straight, grab a power rack or stationary object to brace yourself, and place your left heel in the hole of a weight plate.

Slide the weight as close to your body as possible by bending your knee. (Your right leg stays straight.)

Push the weight back to the starting position, and repeat. Finish all of your repetitions, then switch legs. To emphasize your glutes (that is, your butt), start with your left leg in the same position as before, but bend your right knee and place your right foot flat on the floor. Then lift your hips so your body forms a straight line from shoulder to right knee for the entire move.

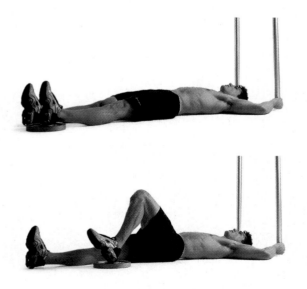

Prepare for Powder

Skiing and snowboarding are sports that require balance and lower-body strength. You'll improve both with this exercise from Andy Walshe, sports-science director for the U.S. Ski Team. This lunge variation builds strength and balance while simulating the motion of skiing as well as riding, says Walshe.

'ROUND-THE-CLOCK LUNGE Stand with your feet hip-width apart, and hold dumbbells at your sides. Step backward with your right leg to six o'clock, until your right knee is just above the floor and your left thigh is parallel to the floor, keeping your left knee over (not past) your toes.

Push back up to the starting position and repeat, this time stepping backward to five o'clock, but keeping your toes pointed straight ahead. Move around the clock, lunging back to four o'clock next, then straight out to the side, then to two o'clock, and so on to 12 o'clock. Now switch legs and step back with your left leg, moving from six o'clock clockwise to 12.

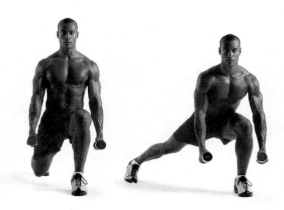

A Cut Above

The key to carving through powder on a snowboard is controlling the toe- and heel-side edges of the board, says Linda Crocket, national education director of the American Association of Snowboard Instructors. When you lean out over the front of your board in a wicked toe-side turn, you need strong, well-developed calves to get farther out on the edge and maintain proper balance. And the faster you fly, the greater the forces will be on those muscles.

Try this combination move from Lisa Wolfe, A.C.E., a trainer in Howell, Michigan.

THE EXPRESS LIFT Hold a pair of dumb-bells just outside your shoulders, with your arms bent and palms facing each other. Stand with your knees slightly bent and the balls of your feet shoulder-width apart on 25-pound weight plates.

Push the weights straight overhead as you raise your heels as high as you can. Pause, then slowly lower the weights and your heels back to the starting position. Do three sets of 8 to 12 repetitions one or two times a week.

PEAK performance

Make Leg Work the Pillar of Your Lifting Program

Norwegian researchers have found that beginning lifters gain upper-body strength by doing lower-body exercises. In the study of 18 men doing both upper- and lower-body exercises, those who emphasized the lower-body work actually gained the most upper-body strength. Your legs have a lot of muscle mass, so when you stress them, you trigger a release of hormones, which in turn stimulates muscle growth throughout your body, explains Wayne Westcott, Ph.D., C.S.C.S., a fitness researcher based in Quincy, Massachusetts. In addition, one of the lower-body exercises used in the study was the squat, which also works much of your upper body. Whether you're just starting out or you're a longtime lifter, make leg work the foundation of your program.

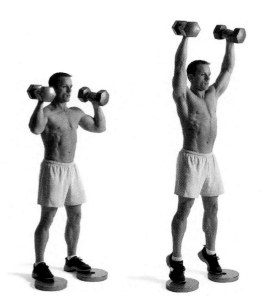

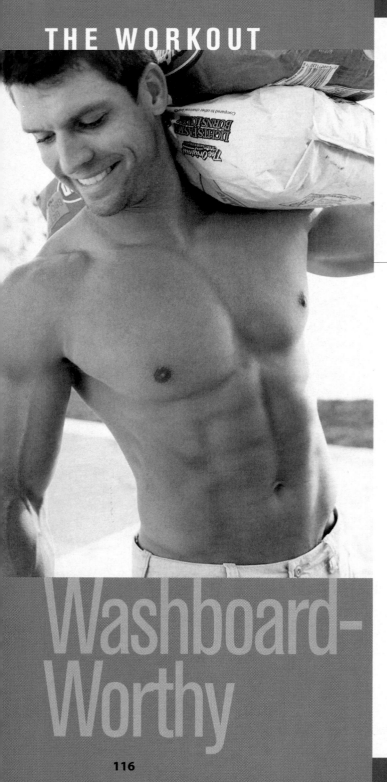

Washboard-Worthy

Find your abs with our 8-week belly-busting plan

You know they're under there somewhere. Your abs, that is. With this gut-busting program, you'll unearth that long lost six-pack in just 8 weeks. So start counting down the days until you can take off your shirt—and leave it off.

Instructions

Most of the exercises in these workouts are the same for both beginner and advanced lifters. The few exceptions are labeled beginner or advanced.

Use the guidelines for the beginner workout if you have less than a year of strength training experience or if you're coming back from a layoff of longer than 4 months. Do the intermediate/advanced program if you've worked out consistently for the past year or longer.

If you belong to a gym, you can do the workouts exactly as they are shown in the next few pages. If you work out at home or have limited equipment, you can perform

BY MICHAEL MEJIA, C.S.C.S.

any of the barbell moves with dumbbells. For exercises that require a cable machine or other gym equipment, we offer an alternative you can do at home with a barbell or dumbbells.

The Workout

Alternate between workout A and workout B, 3 days a week. Rest a day after each workout. You'll perform each exercise in workout A and workout B as either a hybrid exercise or a superset.

Hybrids are combinations of two or more exercises performed as a single move. So, in a hybrid, you'll do one repetition of each combination, then repeat it until you've completed the prescribed number of repetitions for a set of each move. Rest 90 seconds between hybrids.

In supersets—pairs of exercises that work opposite muscle groups—you'll do two different exercises back-to-back, without rest in between. Rest 60 to 90 seconds after each superset. Follow these workout guidelines:

Weeks 1–4 *Hybrids:* Do 2 or 3 sets of 8 to 10 repetitions. *Supersets:* Do 2 or 3 sets of 10 to 12 repetitions

Weeks 5–8 *Hybrids:* Do 2 or 3 sets of 5 to 7 repetitions. *Supersets:* Do 2 or 3 sets of 6 to 8 repetitions

INTERMEDIATE/ADVANCED

Weeks 1–4 *Hybrids:* Do 2 or 3 sets of 5 to 7 repetitions. *Supersets:* Do 2 or 3 sets of 10 to 12 repetitions

Weeks 5–8 *Hybrids:* Do 2 or 3 sets of 3 to 5 repetitions. *Supersets:* Do 2 or 3 sets of 6 to 8 repetitions

Do the abdominal workout as a circuit, performing one set of an exercise after another with no rest in between, before each total-body workout. Do two or three circuits, performing 8 to 12 repetitions of each exercise. Rest 1 to 2 minutes between circuits.

COMPLEX 1: HYBRID

BARBELL POWER CLEAN/FRONT SQUAT/PUSH PRESS

Advanced Start Here

● Squat over a loaded barbell on the floor, and grip it overhand at shoulder width—just as if you were starting a standard deadlift.

Beginner Start Here

● You'll actually be doing a hang clean instead of a power clean. Grab the barbell with a full, overhand, shoulder-width grip. Set your feet shoulder-width apart, with your knees bent about 30 degrees, and bend forward at the hips as you hold the bar at arm's length just above your knees.

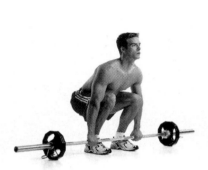

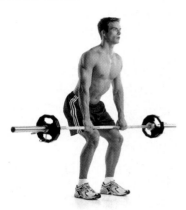

● Pull the bar up from the starting position as fast as you can, go up on your toes, shrug your shoulders, and perform an upright row as you lift the bar up along your body.

● When the bar hits chest level, "catch" it on your front shoulders by dropping under it in a half-squat and turning your palms up toward the ceiling. Your upper arms should be parallel to the floor when the bar lands on your shoulders.

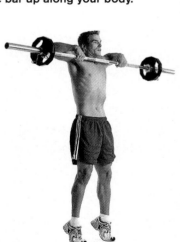

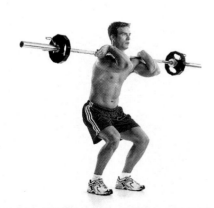

● Initiating the movement from your hips, not your knees, lower yourself as though sitting in a chair behind you. Keeping your elbows as high as you can throughout the move, descend into a full front squat so that your upper thighs are parallel to the floor.

● Drive yourself up with your legs as you thrust the weight toward the ceiling until you are standing upright and your arms are straightened above you, elbows locked. Slowly return to the starting position.

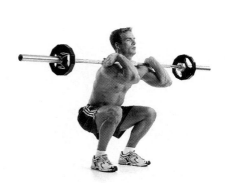

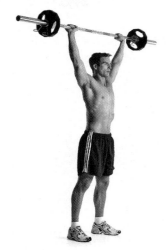

COMPLEX 2: HYBRID

ROMANIAN DEADLIFT/BENT-OVER ROW

● Grab the barbell with an overhand, shoulder-width grip, and stand holding it at arm's length in front of your thighs. Set your feet shoulder-width apart with a very slight bend in your knees. Pull your shoulders back.

● Bend over at the hips to lower the bar down your legs, toward the floor. Stop when your torso is parallel to the floor or when you can't go lower without rounding your back. Keep your knees bent at the same angle and your shoulder blades pulled back throughout.

● With your shoulder blades still pulled back, lift the bar up to the lower part of your sternum (breastbone). Pause at the top, with your chest sticking out toward the bar. Slowly stand up, and lower the bar to the starting position.

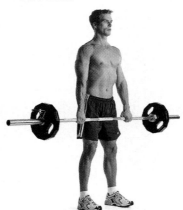

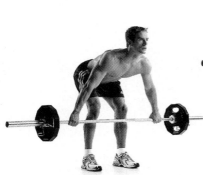

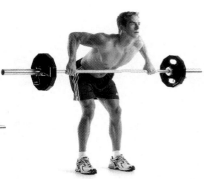

LAT PULLDOWN/BEGINNER (Alternate: Barbell or Dumbbell Pullover)

● Attach the long straight bar to the high cable, and slide a bench underneath it. Sit on the bench, and grab the bar with a false (thumb on the same side as your fingers), overhand, shoulder-width grip. Keep your arms straight and your torso upright or leaning back slightly.

● Pull your shoulder blades together and down, stick your chest out, and pull the bar to your chest. Pause with the bar an inch or two off your chest, then slowly let it rise to the starting position. Keep your chest out.

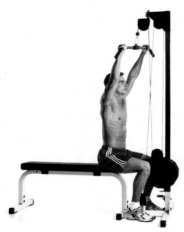
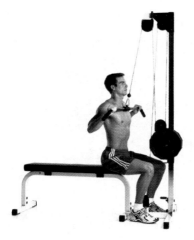

PULLUP/ADVANCED

● Grab a pullup bar with an overhand grip that's slightly wider than shoulder width. Hang with your elbows slightly bent.

● Pull yourself up so that your chin is above the bar. Hold for a second or two, and lower your body with control.

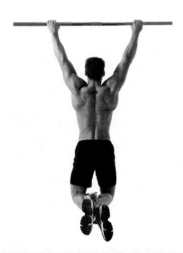
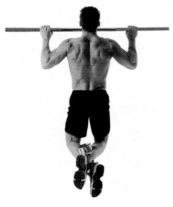

DUMBBELL INCLINE PISTON PRESS

● Set the bench to between 10 and 30 degrees to target your upper chest. Hold two dumbbells with an overhand grip a few inches higher than chest level, so they are right next to your armpits. Keep your shoulder blades pulled back.

● Press one arm straight up over your chest. Pause, then push the other up as you bring the first arm down to the starting position.

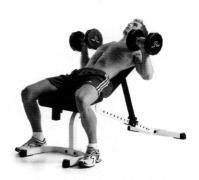

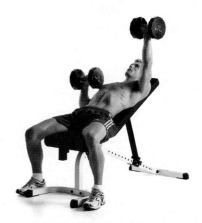

WORKOUT B

COMPLEX 1: HYBRID

BARBELL SPLIT SQUAT/OVERHEAD PRESS

● Grab the barbell in an overhand, shoulder-width grip. Bring your elbows forward so your palms face up. Rest the bar on your front delts. (This is just like the "catch" position of the power clean.) Stand with

one foot 2½ to 3 feet in front of the other, each in line with its corresponding buttock.

● Keep your upper body erect as you descend until the top of your front thigh is parallel to the ground.

● Push through your feet to stand up as you press the bar overhead until your arms are straight with locked elbows. Pause, then lower the bar and return to the starting position.

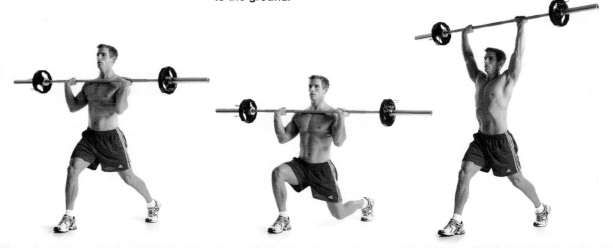

REVERSE PUSHUP

● Secure a bar on a weight rack about 3 feet above the floor. Lie down so the bar is directly over your chest. Grab the bar with an overhand grip that's slightly wider than shoulder width. Lift your torso and legs off the floor, so that only the backs of your heels remain planted. Pull in your abs, and hold your body in a straight line from head to heels.

● Pinch your shoulder blades together as you pull your chest up as close as possible to the bar.

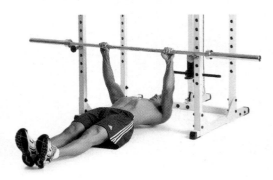 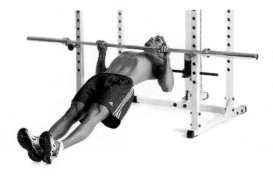

DIP (Alternate: Incline Bench Press)

● Step onto the foot supports of a dip station, grabbing the ends of the handles with a neutral grip. Jump up, and steady yourself. You want to start the movement with your arms straight but not locked, and your body perfectly still. You can cross your legs behind you or leave them hanging straight down.

● Slowly lower yourself until your upper arms are parallel to the floor. (If possible, do this in front of a mirror; going lower is brutal to your shoulders.) Push back up to the starting position.

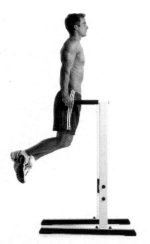 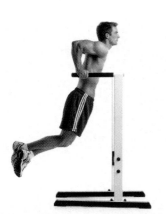

DUMBBELL LUNGE/HAMMER CURL

● Start with your feet hip-width apart, and hold two dumbbells at your sides.

● Take a bold stride forward with your right leg, far enough so that your front thigh ends up parallel to the floor with your knee over (not past) your toes. Quickly push back up to the starting position.

● Without changing your wrist position, slowly curl the weights up toward your shoulders.

Keep your upper arms tucked against your sides throughout. Pause, then lower the weights back to your sides.

● Take a bold stride forward with your left leg, far enough so that your front thigh ends up parallel to the floor with your knee over (not past) your toes. Quickly push back up to the starting position.

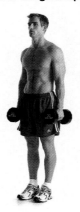
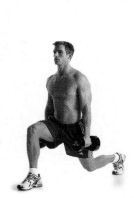
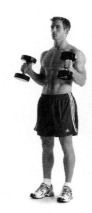
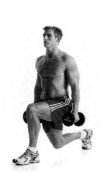

ABDOMINAL WORKOUT

INCLINE REVERSE CRUNCH/BEGINNER

● Lie on an incline bench set at a 45-degree angle, so that your torso and buttocks are on the bench and your legs hang off. Using your abdominal muscles, hold your feet off the floor, keeping your knees slightly bent. To keep your body securely in place throughout the move, reach around and hold onto the bench supports.

● Use your abdominal muscles to crunch your pelvis toward your rib cage. Your tailbone should rise a few inches off the bench as your knees move toward your chin. Pause, then slowly return to the starting position.

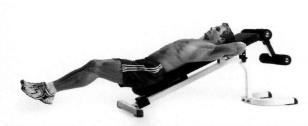
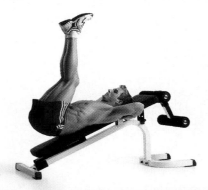

HANGING LEG RAISE/ADVANCED

● Grab a chinup bar with an overhand grip slightly wider than shoulder width, and hang with your knees slightly bent.

● Use the muscles of your lower abs to pull your hips up as you curl them toward your chest. Lift your knees as close to your chest as possible, rounding your lower back. Pause, and feel the contraction in your lower abdominal muscles. Then return to the starting position.

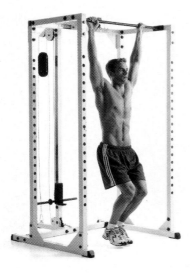
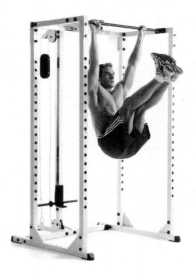

SWISS BALL OBLIQUE CRUNCH (Alternate: Oblique Crunch on the floor)

● Lie sideways on a Swiss ball. Hold your hands behind your ears, and keep your legs straight, feet on the floor. (You can anchor yourself by bracing your feet against a wall.)

● Lift your shoulder, and crunch sideways in a straight line toward your hip. Don't twist. Hold for a second before returning to the starting position.

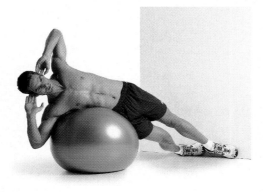
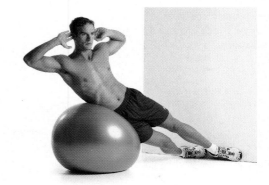

CABLE CRUNCH (Alternate: Weighted Crunch)

● Attach a rope handle to a high pulley. Face the machine, grab the ropes, and kneel in front of the weight stack with your buttocks near your heels but not resting on them. Hold the ropes at the sides of your face with your elbows pointing straight down to the floor.

● Crunch your rib cage toward your pelvis without moving any other part of your lower body from its original position. Pause when your elbows approach your knees, then slowly return to the starting position.

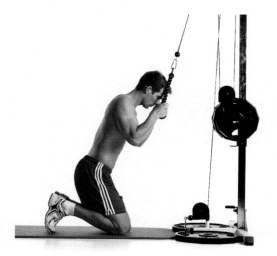 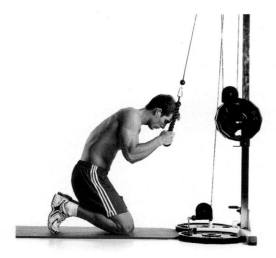

BRIDGE

● On an exercise mat, get into a modified pushup position with your weight on your forearms and toes. Your body should form a straight line from head to heels (don't let your back sag). Pull your abs in as far as you can, and hold this position for 20 to 60 seconds, breathing steadily. Relax before returning to the starting position.

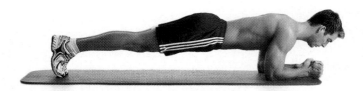

This workout series is adapted from *The Men's Health Home Workout Bible,* by Lou Schuler, with exercise programs by Michael Mejia, M.S., C.S.C.S. © 2002 by Rodale Inc. Available wherever books are sold.

TRAINING TIPS

Q Is there a leg exercise I can do without hitting the weight rack?

A.C., KANSAS CITY, MISSOURI

A Use the weight set your mom gave you: your body. The Bulgarian squat uses your entire body weight to build muscle and keeps the weight on through a greater range of motion than traditional leg exercises, says Ian King, C.S.C.S., owner of King Sports and co-author of *The Book of Muscle*. Besides, Bulgarian squat is a great name to drop. Here's how to do it: Stand 3 feet in front of a bench with your hands on your head. Place your stronger

leg behind you, and rest your other foot on the bench. Lower your body until your front knee is bent 90 degrees and your rear knee nearly touches the floor. Your front lower leg should be perpendicular to the floor, and your torso should remain upright. Take 8 seconds to lower yourself, pause for 1 second, then take 4 seconds to push yourself back to the starting position. Finish all of your repetitions, then repeat the move, this time with your stronger leg forward. As it gets easier, hold dumbbells in your hands or load a bar on your shoulders.

LOOK F-ABULOUS

Sit Up and Take Notice

You can do crunches till you puke, but according to a new study from the Medical College of Georgia, if you're trying to build abs, situps are the best way to get the job done. Researchers at the school had a group of volunteers perform six different ab exercises and electronically monitored their muscle contractions. Here's how the exercises they looked at ranked, from best to worst.

Full situp on the floor ★★★★★★
Full situp using an exercise ball, unassisted ★★★★★
Full situp using an exercise ball, assisted ★★★★
Crunch using an exercise ball, unassisted ★★★
Crunch using an exercise ball, assisted ★★
Crunch on the floor ★

TRI THIS ON FOR SIZE

Q I do every triceps exercise in the book, and mine don't grow. Why?

T.T., RUSTON, LOUISIANA

A Depends on the book. Most focus on exercises with the entire movement in your elbow joint. But triceps are also involved in shoulder action. The biggest part—the long head, on the inside of your upper arm—is mainly involved. At the end of your next upper-body workout, try this long-head-blasting superset: Start with a combination of EZ-curl-bar pullovers and extensions.

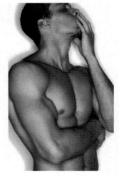

Lie on your back, hold the bar over your nose with straight arms, then bend your elbows and rotate your shoulders as you lower the bar behind your head. Pull it up to the starting position. After 8 to 10 repetitions, set down the bar and pick up dumbbells. Hold them with your palms facing each other. Repeat the set, but don't bend your elbows. Just do straight-arm pullovers. You should find your shirt sleeves getting tighter.

REACH YOUR PEAK

Is there any way to get a better biceps peak?
M.T., SAN BERNADINO, CALIFORNIA

Your biceps shape is mostly genetic. However, you can use a few tricks to bring out whatever peak you're fated to have. And, hey, if your biceps are big enough, no one will notice if they have no peak to speak of.

One exercise that helps with both issues is the prone 45-degree curl. You set an incline bench to a 45-degree angle, lie on your chest on the bench, let your arms hang straight down from your shoulders, and lift dumbbells or an EZ-curl bar. "The angle makes the contraction more intense at the top," says Michael Mejia, C.S.C.S., coauthor of *The Home Workout Bible.*

You get the opposite effect

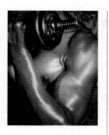

when you do a preacher curl. That exercise is toughest right at the beginning of the movement and much easier at the top, when there's no resistance from gravity. Mejia suggests trying a set of preachers followed immediately by a set of prone curls.

SPORT A SIX-PACK

I'm pretty lean, and I do 50 crunches every day, but there's still no signs of abs underneath my shirt. What can I do?
J.B., KETTERING, OHIO

For starters, stop doing so many crunches. Instead, add weights to your ab routine and bust your gut only three times a week. The result: You'll shock your muscles into growing and give them the downtime necessary to grow forth and multiply (by six). Try this Zercher situp from Mike Gough, C.S.C.S., owner of optperformance.com. Grab an EZ-curl bar (add weight if you can handle more then 25 pounds for 10 repetitions), and hold it in the

crooks of your elbows. Lie on your back, your knees bent and feet flat on the floor.

Slowly lift your torso to a sitting position.

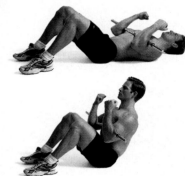

Pause, then slowly lower to the floor. Three days a week, do three or four sets of eight reps with a weight you can lift 10 times at most.

PRESS HERE FOR PECS

What's the best exercise for building definition on the outer edge of the pectorals?
L.J., FALMOUTH, MASSACHUSETTS

If you have definition around the edges, it's because you have little fat there. And if you don't like your outer-chest development, you likely have little bulk in your pectorals overall. Try heavy chest presses to build mass.

OUTRUN
ANYONE

For lots of guys, running is a staple of their exercise routine, partly because it's a great way to stay lean, and partly because it's so simple. Just lace up your Nikes, and head out the door. Plus, the monotony of pounding the pavement can be therapeutic—a time to get away from office politics, de-stress, and take in your surroundings.

Runners are a different breed, a competitive lot. Whether you run alone or with buddies, you're always trying to better your time, or lap the stranger up ahead. This section will have you running long and running strong. Build endurance and beat boredom with new run routines. Increase speed and explosive power to get you out of the blocks fast. And defy the old saying "No pain, no gain" with tips on treating common runner's ailments—and ways to prevent them in the first place.

Speaking of first place, that's where you'll be in your next 10-K. You'll post your best time ever with our patented go-fast plan. Because we never did understand that other old saying, "Save the best for last." Who the heck wants to be last? At least you'll never know what that's like . . .

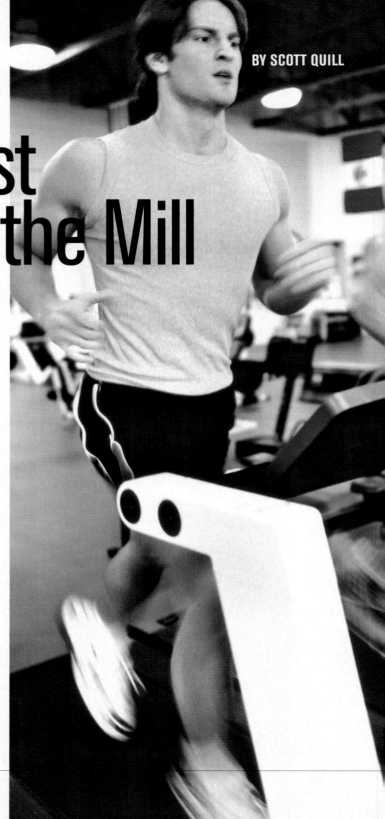

BY SCOTT QUILL

Not Just Run of the Mill

Make your treadmill workouts more fun this winter

Treadmills make me feel like a lab rat: caged in a gym, getting nowhere, with a vague sense that life is pointless. Which got me wondering how scientists keep their clueless little research rodents running on treadmills in their experiments.

Turns out it's Cheerios. Cheerios and a little electrical shock if they slow down.

"It's a very small current. But they don't seem to like it," Steven Britton, Ph.D., a professor of physiology at the Medical College of Ohio, tells me. After a session, he says, he rewards each rat with a Cheerio.

"In Norway," he mentions, "they give them a little piece of chocolate."

Intriguing. But shock therapy isn't going to happen at my gym. And chocolate is part of the sweet holiday minefield that puts me and other men on the treadmill in the first place. Then Britton, being a scientist, makes an intuitive leap: "If people are informed of the consequences of being overweight and not exercising, that's kind of a little shocker."

Eureka! So I, being a journalist, twisted his idea and did some research, making a negative jolt a positive push:

• Men who exercised for 30 minutes on a treadmill boosted their levels of phenylacetic acid—a natural antidepressant—by 77 percent. Perfect for gloomy winter days.

• Running for an hour or more per week reduces your chance of coronary heart disease by 42 percent, according to Harvard researchers.

• Running on a treadmill instead of on roads reduces your chances of a stress fracture by at least 48 percent, a study showed.

Taping these findings to the treadmill's control panel would help. But here are some more practical boredom busters that will make your time on the belt seem to go faster. For all of these, make sure you jog easily for 5 minutes to warm up, jog another 5 to cool down, and stretch afterward.

Then go ahead, have a Cheerio.

Mix it up with incline intervals. The term "intervals" usually means a series of short, hard runs interspersed with jogging or

Buying a Treadmill

Dress properly when you shop for a treadmill: running shoes, shorts, and shirt. Expect to pay $1,500 to $3,000 for a sturdy, dependable machine. For that money, you must try it out—extensively. The best brands in that range—such as PaceMaster, True, Landice, LifeFitness, and Precor—are found at specialty fitness stores. Bring your senses:

Touch. Go for a serious test run, changing speeds and in-clines several times. You're going to spend hours on this thing; surely you can spare 20 minutes for a tryout. "Trust your instincts—go with what feels best," says Dave Sellers, former new-product editor for *Runner's World.* You want a solid deck, good cushioning, and a responsive motor. "If it feels like junk," says Sellers, "it probably is."

Sight. Look at the display and the controls. "Find the balance between abundant features and simplicity that suits you," Sellers says. If the controls are too confusing, move on. You'll spend a lot of time pushing buttons and looking at numbers, so you should be comfortable with them.

Hearing. Rattling handrails, a straining motor, and a deck so noisy it'll wake the kids are warning signs of poor quality.

walking. In this variation, instead of speeding up for the hard stints, you increase the incline. The high level of effort will improve your power, says Tony Veney, a track coach at UCLA. Here's how: Set the treadmill's speed for about half of your full effort. Set the incline at 3 percent, run for 20 to 30 seconds, then return to a zero incline for 30 seconds. Repeat this sequence at 5 percent, and then 7 percent. That's one repetition. Do 8 to 10 repetitions.

Try TV time-outs. If there's a television in your gym (or basement), use it to time your "pickups" (sustained intervals in which you pick up the pace), suggests Budd Coates, a four-time qualifier for the Olympic Marathon trials and special contributor to

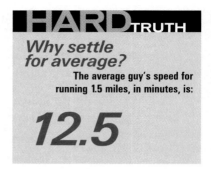

HARD TRUTH

Why settle for average?

The average guy's speed for running 1.5 miles, in minutes, is:

12.5

Runner's World magazine. Say you're watching a basketball game. Whenever the clock stops (time-outs, foul shots), bump up your pace to about 80 percent effort. When the game's in progress, dial down to a jog. It works with any sport or any TV show. Run hard during Katie's segments; jog during Matt's. Or, when Bill O'Reilly gets rude, pick up the pace; when he's being civil, jog. (Warning: You need to be in good shape for this one.)

Take a shot at negative splits. No, this doesn't refer to an uptight cheerleader. This concept burns fat, makes the time fly, and will help you in your next race. "Negative splits" means you're running faster at the end than at the start. In this session, start at a jog, and at every quarter mile, punch the speed button one beep higher. (You can do this for any length interval.) Push this as long as you like, but give yourself a smooth cooldown. Breaking the run into chunks makes it less tedious, and training your body to start slow and end fast will pay off next time you're in a road race; you'll hold back at the start when your adrenaline is high, and finish strong when others fade.

Live on the edge. This goes against all those lawyers' warnings, but it works for David Deubelbeiss, the Boss of the Belt. He's a Toronto ultramarathoner who set a world record by running 130.82 miles on a treadmill in 24 hours. (And who knows boredom better than a Canadian?) His tip:

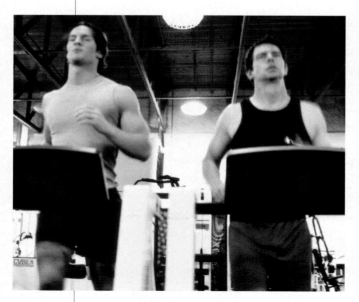

Peek Performance

You're not alone if you compete with your treadmill neighbor

BY KEVIN COOK

I admit it—I peek. Here I am, almost shoulder-to-shoulder with the next guy at the health club, sneaking a glance. I don't want him to catch me, so I wait until he's looking straight ahead. Then I peek. And it's about what I expected: 7.5 miles per hour. Until the SOB reaches down and punches it up to 8.

I never planned to be a treadmill racer. In fact, I came inside to escape a similar event: the jogging-path ego race. At age 40, scared by a cholesterol test and a doctor who wanted to put me on prescription drugs for life, I started running. It was awful at first, but I stuck with it, and it soon became a daily pleasure that flushed the Crisco from my veins and cured my desk-job lethargy. But the more I ran, the more I got into brief competitions, speeding up to pass the runner ahead of me, and then the one ahead of him. This can be rationalized: Following another guy's butt for 4 miles doesn't appeal to me. But some guys—never women, who seem to be immune to such alpha-chimp tactics—fought back, picking up their paces to keep me from passing. A minute later we'd be running hard, looking straight ahead, pretending we'd just happened to shift into turbo at the same instant, until one of us saved face by peeling off down a side street.

Joining a health club was supposed to end those exhausting mini-machothons. It didn't. At the club, I find myself locked in a grudge race with the guy beside me at least once a week. We eventually beep our speed up to 9 mph. At that point, victory can be measured in tenths. Keep up a 9.4-mph pace to the other's 9.3 until he backs off or steps off, and it's your day.

A recent lunchtime workout wasn't any different. The other guy was a few years younger, but not enough to matter. We both wore plain shorts and T-shirts, signaling our no-nonsense approach to the task at hand, which started at an easy 6 mph for me—and 6.5 for him (I peeked). Half an hour later, we were both at 8, having logged about 3¼ miles each. I went up to 9, and he answered. At the 35-minute mark, we were matching strides at 10. With no more speed in the machines, this was now an endurance race. Who would quit first? Neither of us acknowledged the race we were running. And I had long since forgotten a business meeting I was supposed to make.

Three minutes later, my eyes watering, I punched the stop button. Conceding defeat, I grabbed a towel, mopped my sopping brow, and went for a shower. As I washed off the sweat, I felt like a loser, but the feeling passed. Getting dressed, remembering the business meeting, I was Button-Down Man again. That's when I bumped into my foe.

We were going out the front door, thinking of other things, when we almost collided.

"Oh, sorry."

"Excuse me."

We stood still. Some male code mandated that we pretend nothing had happened, though our little race might be the most intense confrontation either of us would have that week. For 45 minutes we had been athletes; now we were men in ties, wondering what to say.

We said the right thing: nothing. He nodded. So did I. Then he went left, and I went right.

When you get bored, slow your stride (not the speed of the treadmill) so you drift toward the back edge of the belt. When your heels touch the end, quickly step up to the front. Do this at a relatively slow belt speed, warns Deubelbeiss, and don't try it until you can run without looking at any part of the treadmill for 30 seconds.

Crest that hill. This drill from Jane Hahn, a senior editor at *Runner's World,* will help you run hills effectively, attacking the slope and exploding over the top. It'll also help you put on bursts of speed on the flat. Run for 3 minutes at a 3 percent incline, then flatten it out and maintain the same level of effort by speeding up the belt a few notches for 1 minute. Recover with a minute of jogging, then repeat the sequence three times.

Power up the tunes! Load your MP3 player wisely. A British study found that men can handle much higher workloads when listening to music that builds in tempo from slow to fast, rather than maintaining a consistently fast beat. So start out slow with Coldplay, mix in some White Stripes, and end with the Ramones. A great runner's player is the tiny iRiver iFP-390T. It holds up to 8 hours of music, has an FM tuner and a voice recorder, and straps to your arm. $200, bestbuy.com

Watch yourself. Use your club's mirrors for something other than checking out the redhead wearing the Under Armour. Look at yourself occasionally, especially when running fast. "Monitoring your stride mechanics gives you something to concentrate on, and you'll run more efficiently," says Bob Larsen, coach of the USA men's distance runners for the 2004 Olympics. Larsen's checklist: (1) Minimize your contact with the belt. Don't bounce; think quick feet. (2) Stand tall, so all your body segments are aligned. (3) Stay loose and relaxed.

Use a heart-rate monitor. If you're bored with the readouts on the treadmill, add another source of input: a heart-rate monitor. "You should train at 60 to 80 percent of your maximum heart rate, because as you exceed 80 percent, results do not increase proportionally to your work," says Richard Stein, M.D., a spokesman for the American Heart Association. See how inclines affect your rate, and notice how quickly your heart recovers from a burst of effort. A terrific new monitor is the Nike Triax Elite. $300, hdosport.com

PEAK
performance

Drink Up

If you're training for an intense race, you may need more than a standard sports drink. According to a new study from the University of Texas, a high-carbohydrate sports drink with a four-to-one ratio of carbs to protein may be the best option for

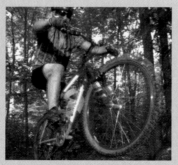

recovering from intense, long-term aerobic activity. In trials, cyclists who drank a high-carb sports drink following a 2-hour ride were able to pedal 55 percent longer before reaching exhaustion than men who drank a standard, lower-carb sports drink.

BY ED EYESTONE

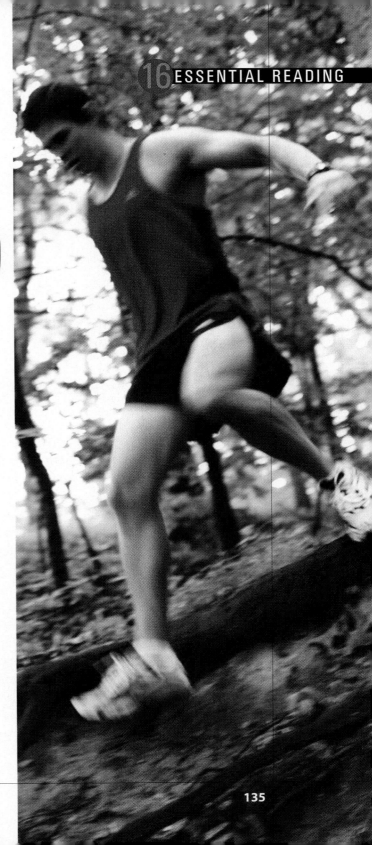

Pick Up the Tempo

8 world-class ways to beat boredom, boost endurance, and run faster

As a two-time Olympic marathoner, I can testify: Running can be boring. And frustrating. Especially the way the typical guy does it—the same 4- or 5-mile jog, day after day, week after week, year after year. Then along comes some race for some cure, and ponytailed old dudes and even a few thirtysomething moms pass him.

The problem: monotonous runs. The simple fix: Go faster once in a while. Read on, and I'll show you how to mix speed into your workouts, shake the boredom from your usual loop, and build your endurance to an all-time high. You'll use the same cutting-edge techniques I use to train the Brigham Young cross-country team. (And myself.)

Don't worry, your regular miles aren't useless. You're burning calories—and burning off stress—while toughening the connective tissues you'll need for my plan. To get started, perform one of these workouts once a week in place of your routine run. Add a second one per week when you're comfortable.

Once you've become a speed freak, here's a great training mix: Do one of the first three workouts early in the week, then choose a second from numbers 4 through 7 later in the week, at the track. Do the last run on the weekend. You'll feel the difference as you start to pass runners in the 9th K of a 10-K, and you'll see the results in bright numbers on the finish-line timer.

1. Tempo Run

What: A fuel-injected version of your 4-mile jog, run at a "comfortably hard" pace.

Why: Tempo runs train your body to clear the lactic acid that causes your muscles to "burn," forcing you to slow down. Everyone has a threshold at which blood lactate dramatically increases. Tempo runs push back your lactate threshold.

How: Estimate your fastest 3-mile time (think back to your best recent 5-K). Calculate the pace per mile, and add 30 seconds to it. So if you think the fastest you can run 3 miles is 24 minutes—that's an 8-minute pace—try for a tempo pace of

Intervals with Iron

Use this concept in the weight room for more power

What can a skinny runner in short shorts teach a weight lifter? Plenty. Interval training translates to the gym. Alternating between light and heavy weights can improve performance in all sports, whether it's a torqued-up softball swing or a faster fast break.

Using light weight allows you to accelerate through a lift, and that helps build power; a couple of good examples are jump-squats and bench-press throws (in which you release the weight at the top of the lift in a Smith machine).

A study published in the *Journal of Strength and Conditioning Research* found that lifters who added a heavy set of bench presses between light sets of bench-press throws generated 4.5 percent more power in the bench-press throws than those who didn't do the heavy bench presses in between.

"Heavy resistances stiffen your muscles and increase neural activity," says Daniel Baker, C.S.C.S., the lead study author. In other words, your muscles learn to manage heavy weight and then move with in-creased velocity when the load is lightened; your brain prepares your muscles to lift a heavy load even after the weight is reduced.

Baker recommends using a weight that's 65 percent of your one-rep maximum—the most you can lift no more than one time—for the heavy sets. Try doing a heavy set of squats before a set of vertical jumps or a light set of jump-squats. No Smith machine? Do a set of bench presses between sets of plyometric pushups, in which you explode off the ground and your hands leave the floor.

8 minutes, 30 seconds per mile for your 4-mile run.

Tip: Be precise. Wear a watch.

2. Tempo 1,000s

What: A series of 1,000-meter runs at your tempo pace, with rest in between.

Why: Short tempo runs help you maintain a strict pace, and the brief recoveries keep you at lactate threshold. Tempo 1,000s are also great if you can't do lengthy tempo runs.

How: Run at tempo pace for 1,000 meters (that's about $2^1/_2$ times around a track), then rest for 60 seconds before repeating. Start with a total of six 1,000-meter intervals and progress to 10, adding one each time you perform the workout.

Tip: If you'd prefer, measure in time instead of distance. Perform each interval for $3^1/_2$ minutes before resting.

3. Step-Down Fartlek

What: "Fartlek" is Swedish for "speed play," meaning you accelerate and slow down according to how you feel. (How European!)

Why: In a step-down fartlek, the intervals are more structured (how American!) and become harder at the end of your run. Working hard when you're tired will make you faster when you're fresh.

How: Start at a pace that's about 75 percent of your full effort, and go for 5 minutes. Then slow down to about 40 percent effort for 5 minutes. Continue this fast-then-slow pattern, but shorten the hard-running segment by a minute each time while in-

PAINkiller

In Stitches
How do I get rid of a side stitch?

D.R., San Mateo, California

No one's sure what causes these sharp pains under the rib cage, though it could be either the diaphragm (your breathing muscle) or trapped gas pockets from a full stomach. Try this stretch: Raise your right arm, and bend your trunk to the left. Hold for 30 seconds, then stretch the other side. Ed Eyestone, a *Runner's World* columnist and Olympic marathoner, recommends tightening your abdominal muscles, rubbing out the pain with your fingers, or exhaling forcefully as the foot opposite the stitch hits the ground. One more thing: Don't eat and run. Give your body time, ideally 2 to 3 hours, to digest, and avoid foods high in sugar or fat.

creasing your speed. By the last 1-minute burst, you should be almost sprinting.

Tip: Each week, add 1 minute to your first segment—but keep doing the same step-down sequence—until your first interval is 10 minutes.

4. Mile Repeats

What: Hard 1-mile runs with rest in between. The ultimate training tool for the serious runner.

Why: The length and intensity of mile repeats force you to work at the edge of your aerobic limit, giving you the endurance and mental toughness you need to run hard for long periods of time.

How: Run three or four 1-mile intervals at your 5-K race pace. After each mile, rest for 4 minutes.

Tip: Budget your effort so that you run each quarter mile at the same pace.

5. 800 Repeats

What: Hard runs with jogging recoveries.

Why: Running at your maximum aerobic capacity is the best way to improve it. The payoff: You'll be able to run faster with the same effort.

How: Warm up until you're sweating. Subtract 10 seconds from your mile-repeat pace, and maintain that speed for 800 meters (twice around the track). After each 800-meter run, jog once around the track before repeating.

Tip: Start with only four intervals per session, and add one each workout until you can comfortably do eight.

6. 400 Repeats

What: Really hard runs with jogging recoveries.

Why: You'll develop the fast-twitch muscles you need to finish strong. Fast-twitch fibers also give you the strength and power to run faster with less effort.

How: Run at your fastest 1-mile pace. (So if your personal record, or PR, for the mile is 7 minutes, you'll want to perform each 400-meter interval in 105 seconds, or 1:45.) After each 400-meter run, jog for 1 or 2 minutes, then repeat. Start with a six-interval workout, and add one each time you go to the track, until you reach 10.

Tip: Do the math before you start. And warm up first!

7. In-and-Outs

What: Fast 200-meter runs alternating with not-so-fast 200-meter runs for 2 miles total.

Why: This workout forces you to recover on the go, allowing you to train at higher overall intensity for a longer distance than you otherwise could.

How: At your mile PR pace, run 200 meters, then slow down so it takes you 10 seconds longer to complete the next 200 meters. Continue to alternate between these speeds until you've run 2 miles.

Tip: If you slow by more than 2 seconds in either your fast or slow segment, run at a light pace until you finish the entire 2 miles.

8. Fast-Finish Long Run

What: A long run with a speed surge in the second half.

Why: You'll train your body to go long and finish strong. And your shorter runs will seem easier.

How: Double your regular easy run. Do the first half at your normal pace, and at the midway point pick up the pace by 5 to 10 seconds per mile.

Tip: Carry water to help you in that second half.

Speed Things Up

Tom Shaw, speed coach for the New England Patriots, swears he can make any man faster. Even you

If you're like most guys, you associate explosiveness more with your digestive system than with your leg muscles. Although speed may have been something you had when you were younger, it's far down your list of fitness priorities now. No doubt you've accepted the fact that you'll never again be cat-quick, and you've learned to compensate.

Shame on you, says Tom Shaw. At age 43, he can still clock 4.65 seconds in the 40-yard dash, which is fast enough to humble some of the bigger running backs in the NFL. Shaw is also a strength-and-conditioning coach, specializing in speed development, for the New England Patriots. Recognize any of these names? Peyton Manning, Tom Brady, Michael Vick, Jeremiah Trotter, Darren Sharper, Shawn Barber, Ricky Williams, Warrick Dunn, Deion Sanders, Rod Woodson, Terrell Buckley . . . Over the years, Shaw has worked with all these guys, plus hundreds of other elite athletes.

"I can make anyone faster," he says matter-of-factly. "If you train properly, get rid of wasted movement, and work on explosiveness, you can increase your speed regardless of age or genetics."

We caught up with Shaw at the Patriots' training camp in Foxboro, Massachusetts, where he promises new players he can train them to cover 40 yards at least two-tenths of a second faster than they ever have before. In the NFL, that's equivalent to 3 yards, which can make the difference between success and failure in breaking (or making) tackles. If Shaw can significantly improve the performance of already finely honed athletes, imagine what he can do for a dull blade like you. And in case you're thinking explosiveness isn't something your sport requires, think again. Whether you swing a golf club or a softball bat, shoot a basketball or a rapid, move a barbell or a mountain bike, if you can do it quicker and with more authority and power, you'll do it better. There are other advantages, too.

You'll build muscle. Sprinting and explosive conditioning are forms of strength training.

You'll lose fat. Interval training—another name for speed training—is a proven fat burner. Plus, the more explosive muscle you build, the more fat you'll burn every second of the day.

You'll stay injury-free. It's the quick bursts (jumping for a rebound, accelerating away from home plate) that cripple weekend warriors. All the more reason to condition these muscles now.

You'll beat boredom. Men abandon exercise programs because there isn't enough variety to hold their attention. This approach supplies plenty of it.

You'll live longer. According to a Harvard study, the more vigorous the activity, the lower the risk of heart disease. Even bursts of 15 minutes help.

You'll look fitter. A sprinter's physique is among the most envied in sport.

You'll save time. Didn't you hear us? It's called speed training.

We've rounded up Shaw's best drills and devices for enhancing speed and explosiveness. It's not so much a program as it is an addendum to whatever you're doing now. Tack a few exercises onto the beginning or end of your regular workout, or make one training day each week a speed day, and see if you don't start experiencing the most important benefit of all: gaining a step and a half on the man you used to be.

Become a Coiled Spring
An NFL wide receiver in full sprint has a ground-contact time of just 0.1 second per

stride. Likewise, an offensive lineman has only 0.25 second to create the momentum for a drive block, and a linebacker just 0.2 second to extend his legs to execute a tackle. Shaw knows; he's done the measurements. And he uses them to impress upon athletes what coiled springs they must be. All that power, all that speed, summoned in a fraction of a second. Unlike in the weight room, where muscles have plenty of time to contract and extend, on the playing field they must operate with hair triggers. Here are some drills designed to develop these characteristics. (Note: Always warm up well and stretch before attempting any of these exercises.)

REACTION/ACCELERATION

Ground starts. Lie facedown. On a starter's command, jump to your feet and sprint all-out for 10 yards. Walk back, and repeat three to five times. "This drill teaches you to stay low and forward and get good thrust," says Shaw.

Pushup starts. Assume a fingertip pushup position. On a starter's command, drive out, staying low, with your shoulders well in front of your hips. Your body angle should be 30 to 40 degrees from vertical at takeoff. Walk back, and repeat three to five times. "This drill makes you take fast-driving steps to keep from falling," says Shaw.

Ball-drop starts. Have a buddy hold a tennis ball in each hand while standing 5 to 10 yards away from you. Assume a down stance, then sprint to whichever ball is

dropped, trying to catch it before it hits the ground a second time. Repeat five to eight times.

EXPLOSIVE POWER

Double-leg vertical jumps. From a standing, one-quarter-squat position, jump forward, bringing both knees toward your chest and keeping your feet together. Repeat continuously for 20 to 30 yards.

Depth jumps. Step off a 20- to 28-inch-high box or stair, then jump up as high as possible. "Quickness off the ground is the key to this drill," says Shaw. "React like a Superball." Repeat five to eight times.

Dumbbell jumps. Hold a light dumbbell (no more than 20 pounds) in each hand. Squat until your thighs are parallel to the ground, then jump as high as possible. Repeat five times. Put down the dumbbells, and do five more jumps.

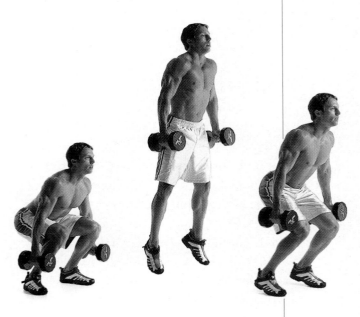

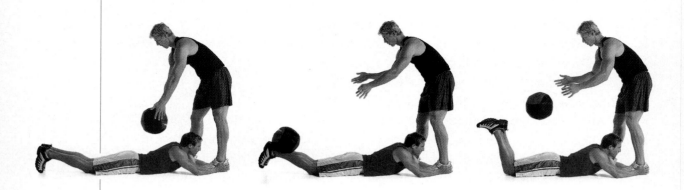

Stadium steps. Find a set of stadium stairs and walk to the top, keeping your steps long and deliberate, with the back leg straight. When this gets too easy, put a sandbag (of reasonable size) on each shoulder.

Roll kicks. For this exercise, you'll need a partner and an oversize ball. Lie facedown with your legs extended. Have your buddy stand in front of your shoulders and roll the ball down your legs. Use your heels to kick it back to him. (Grab his ankle for leverage.) "It's a great way to work the hamstrings, especially when they're fatigued," says Shaw.

QUICKNESS/AGILITY

Take a can of water-based spray paint to the backyard, and draw a ladder of 10 successive 18-inch squares. This is your dance floor.

Run-throughs. From a standing start, run through the ladder, putting one foot in each box. Lift each heel higher than the opposite knee. Turn around at the end, and repeat six to eight times. Catch your breath, then do the same drill but put two feet in each box.

Laterals. Do the ladder sideways by hopping. For the first set of six to eight,

put one foot in each box. For the second set, put two feet in each.

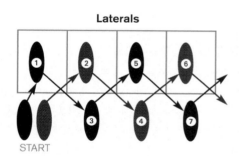

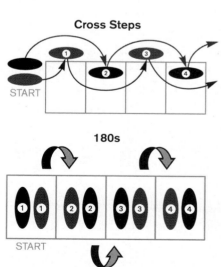

Cross steps. Run along one rail of the ladder, crossing one foot over the other. Turn around; repeat six to eight times.

180s. Face the ladder from the side, step into the first box with both feet, then jump and turn 180 degrees into the next box. Repeat as shown. Do the drill as quickly as possible, four to six times.

POSITION-SPECIFIC SPEEDWORK

To excel at a sport, you must practice its idiosyncratic moves. Shaw calls this "metabolic conditioning," and it involves simulating actual game maneuvers. For instance, he'll have a wide receiver run different pass routes for 2 minutes, take a brief rest, then repeat the sequence. Next to catching balls in a real game, it's the best, most realistic type of conditioning. Use the same logic to devise a workout that's specific to your sport.

Basketball metabolics. For this drill, you'll need a partner to rebound for you. Start by taking a shot from the corner of the baseline, then sprint to the opposite corner and take another shot. Continue back and forth until you make three. Then move to the wing, take a shot, run around the top of the key to the other wing, and shoot again. Continue back and forth until you drop three shots. Then move to the corner of the foul line, shoot, move to the opposite corner, shoot, and continue until you sink three. Finally, shoot from the top of the key. If you miss, sprint to half-court and back, then shoot again. Continue until you sink three shots. As your jumper and endurance improve, increase the number of shots you need to make to move on.

Run like Forrest Gump. Speed requires efficiency. "If you're wasting movement," says Shaw, "you're wasting seconds." A good model, believe it or not, is Tom Hanks as Forrest Gump. The series of photos below showcases some key elements of proper sprinting technique. In fact, just visualizing this scene as you try to run faster will help you cover more ground.

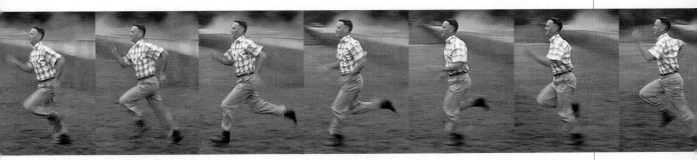

Note Gump's body lean, his hand motion, and where his feet land. This is how you should look (minus the plaid shirt).

Leg action: "Every efficient working machine operates in a circular fashion," says Shaw. "Your legs are no different." Land on the balls of your feet and roll to the toes, keeping a 4- to 6-inch forward lean. Your heels should never touch the ground and, when elevated, should be close to the butt.

Arm action: "Make sure your hands come over your shoulders and behind your hips," says Shaw. Keep your arms bent 90 to 100 degrees, and don't clench your fists. (It

---

Flight Gear

Two products used by the NFL that'll get you ready for takeoff

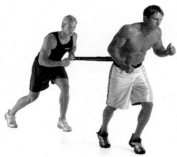

Bullet-Belt Pop and Rip

This device develops explosive power, specifically your first step and the top gear you used to be able to shift into before your clutch blew. It uses an ingeniously simple principle called "pop training." The athlete (yes, that's you) attaches the belt around his waist while a partner stands behind him and grips the handles. From an up or down stance, you drive out and sprint as hard as possible, while your buddy trails behind providing some resistance.

After 10 yards, he pulls one of the cords to release the belt, and you experience an explosive burst that makes it feel as if afterburners have kicked in. The effect is physical as well as psychological. $75. (800) 443-8946, www.bulletbelt.com

Just Jump

This 27-pound, 26-inch-square mat measures vertical leap and leg power. A handheld computer attached to the unit automatically calculates ground time, air time, and the power generated to sky that high. It's fascinating to get a baseline

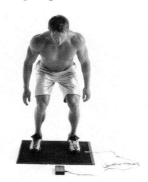

and then see improvement as you do some of the explosive power drills in this chapter. The mat can also be used to gauge reaction time and to time sprints. More fun at parties than Twister. $450. (256) 883-2723; e-mail: mackovja@bellsouth.net

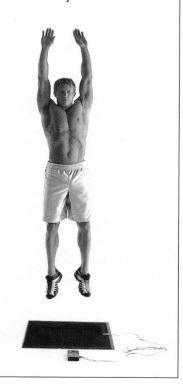

causes muscle tension.) The faster you swing your arms, the faster your legs move. Skeptical? Jog in place, then accelerate arm movement. Your legs will automatically follow.

Stride length: This is the distance traveled with each step. To measure yours, have someone count the number of times your right foot strikes the ground during a 40-yard sprint. For perspective, Deion Sanders needed slightly less than 12 steps to cover 20 yards and just over 18 steps to smoke the entire 40 (time: 4.18 seconds). "Don't make the common mistake of reaching out with your foreleg prior to the foot striking the ground," says Shaw. "This lands the foot well ahead of the knee and brakes your momentum."

One of the quickest and easiest ways to learn proper form is to videotape your workout. Look for flaws in your sprinting technique by viewing it in slow motion and then comparing yourself with Forrest.

Newspaper drills. Here's a great exercise for improving stride length and frequency, the two most important components of running faster. Place rolled-up newspapers (or spray-paint the grass) at steadily lengthening intervals across 40 yards. The first papers should be separated 18 inches, the last ones by 8 feet. Try running alongside, taking only one step at each.

Man makers. You're not going to get fast unless you have sprinter's stamina. Here's a simple but tough workout used by pro football players and other elite athletes to build endurance and burn fat. At first, don't be concerned about time. Just focus on maintaining proper form and completing the

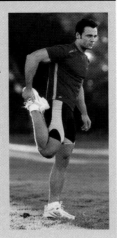

PAINkiller

Shin and Bear It
My shin is killing me. Is this what they call shinsplints?
T.J., Manayunk, Pennsylvania

First, make sure it's not a stress fracture, which is an incomplete crack in the bone. Press your fingers along the shin. A specific spot of pain suggests a fracture. Go to a doctor. Another clue: A fracture may feel okay in the morning, after a rest. Shinsplints, which indicate inflammation, tend to flare in the morning after a night of tightening up, and the pain is more general. Rest, stretching, new shoes, and a softer running surface will relieve shinsplint pain.

workout. As you build endurance, begin abiding by the recommended times. For accuracy (and motivation), do it on a high-school football field.

- Warmup (10-minute jog/stretch)

- 10 100s (100-yard sprints in 15 to 18 seconds, interspersed with 30- to 35-second rests)

- Eight 80s (80-yard sprints in 11 to 15 seconds, with 20- to 25-second rests)

- Six 60s (60-yard sprints in 8 to 11 seconds, with 15- to 20-second rests)

- Four 40s (40-yard sprints in 5 to 8 seconds, with 10- to 15-second rests)

- Cooldown (10-minute jog/stretch)

Tom Shaw conducts 4-day, $450 speed camps in New Orleans. For additional information, call (504) 443-5152 or visit www.coachtomshaw.com.

BY LEN KRAVITZ, PH.D.

Beat the Competition

Kick tail in your next 10-K with our 8-week speed plan

Francis Bellamy can help you run faster than ever before. He's not an Olympic coach or a genetic engineer. He *was* a Baptist minister, born in 1855, who probably never even heard of a 10-K. But in between sermons and baptisms, Bellamy created the ultimate training tool for runners: the Pledge of Allegiance.

No doubt, the ACLU will say this training approach has "vast conspiracy engineered by right-wing joggers" written all over it. Let 'em sue. In a study from the University of Wisconsin at Lacrosse, researchers found that a person's ability to recite the Pledge of Allegiance—all 31 words, out loud—while running is a highly accurate gauge of his intensity of exertion. "It allows you to run at the ideal pace for every single workout, whether it's a long, easy run or high-intensity intervals," says Derek Marks, Ph.D., a professor of human performance at California State University at Stanislaus. And that type of precision training is the key to upgrading your performance and downsizing your race times.

Put it to the test with our patented go-fast plan. We'll show you how reciting on the run can help you turn in your best 10-K time ever. Just one thing: Your right hand? Don't place it over your chest during a race; someone's likely to mistake your patriotism for a heart attack.

The Science of Speed

Before we get to the Pledge, a lesson in lactate threshold. Lactate is your body's buffering agent for the acid that builds up in your legs and causes them to burn during a run. The faster you run, the faster your acid levels rise. At a certain point, there's too much acid to neutralize, and you have to slow down. This is when you've crossed your lactate threshold.

You can also think of your lactate threshold as the fastest pace you can run that allows you to start and finish at the same speed, without feeling any burn. "By pushing your lactate threshold higher, you'll be able to run faster longer," says Ed Coyle,

The Finishing Touches

Boost your workout dividends with these postrun bonus moves

Some guys cap off a run by collapsing. Others hit the shower. You? You're going to squeeze in the exercise equivalent of a "quickie"—that is, 5 minutes of work for an explosive payoff. Here are three results-oriented extras, courtesy of Craig Ballantyne, C.S.C.S., owner of workoutmanuals.com.

Jump higher. Tuck jumps can help even the most earthbound among us elevate our game. Never tuck jumped? Here's how: Jump as high as

you can and bring your knees to your chest (the tuck), then release. When your feet touch the ground, immediately jump again and repeat. Do three sets of six jumps.

Lift more. Get a grip—a strong one—and you'll be able to crank out more pullups and heavier deadlifts. Grab a dumbbell in each hand, let your arms hang naturally at your sides, and walk across the room. For your first set, use heavy dumbbells that allow you to walk for only 20 seconds. Switch to lighter dumbbells for

the next two sets, so you can walk for 40 to 60 seconds, respectively. Rest 1 minute after each set.

Look bigger. A runner with big biceps? It's possible, thanks to down-the-rack training. Choose a weight you can curl eight times at most, and do six to eight repetitions. Immediately grab the next lightest pair of dumbbells, and repeat. Then drop the weight down one more notch, and do as many repetitions as you can.

Ph.D., a professor of kinesiology and health education at the University of Texas. That's where the Pledge of Allegiance comes in: It's the tool that will help you raise your threshold.

Training Days

In this program, you'll run 3 or 4 days a week, usually resting a day after each run. You'll vary the distance and intensity of the workouts, with each designed to build on the preceding one. Follow the guidelines below for performing each workout at the ideal intensity.

Volume training. On volume days, you have just one goal: Log the miles. "Volume training is designed to develop your cardiovascular system's ability to perform prolonged exercise, as well as to prepare your muscles and joints for the repeated impact of running," says Marks.

Intensity: Run at a pace that allows you to recite the Pledge of Allegiance easily.

Maximal steady-state training. You'll perform these runs as close to your lactate threshold as possible. "Maximal steady-state

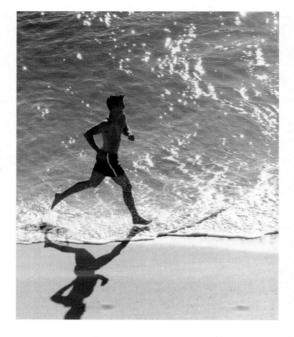

training simulates race pace and improves your body's ability to clear speed-limiting acid from your blood and muscles," says Jerry Mayo, Ph.D., an exercise scientist at Hendrix College in Conway, Arkansas.

Intensity: Run at a pace that allows you to recite the Pledge of Allegiance with difficulty, in spurts of only three or four words at a time.

Interval training. You'll intersperse short bouts of running that are above your lactate threshold with longer periods of running that fall below it. "Intervals train your body to tolerate high amounts of acid," says Marks.

Intensity: Start by running at your volume-training intensity for 5 minutes. Then increase your speed until you can't recite a single word of the Pledge. Maintain this pace for 30 seconds, then slow down to your starting pace for the next 3 minutes, before beginning another 30-second high-intensity stint. Start with five intervals and try to do more each workout, while shortening the duration of the recovery periods.

The Multilevel 10-K Plan

Determine which program is appropriate for your level of fitness, then use the chart below as a guide for your day-by-day workout calendar. Next to each mileage amount is a corresponding letter that indicates whether you perform volume training (V), maximal steady-state training (M), or interval training (I) that day. Complete the entire plan, then repeat it to continue to push your fitness level higher.

Beginner: Follow the beginner program if you perform aerobic exercise or sports 2 or 3 days a week or more.

Advanced: Do the advanced plan if you run at least 20 minutes or 2 miles 3 days a week.

		MONDAY	TUESDAY	WEDNESDAY	THURSDAY	FRIDAY	SATURDAY	SUNDAY
WEEK 1	Beginner	2 miles (V)	Rest	2.5 miles (V)	Rest	3 miles (V)	Rest	3.5 miles (V)
	Advanced	3 miles (V)	Rest	3.5 miles (V)	Rest	4 miles (V)	Rest	4.5 miles (V)
WEEK 2	Beginner	Rest	4 miles (V)	Rest	4 miles (V)	Rest	4 miles (V)	Rest
	Advanced	Rest	5 miles (V)	Rest	5 miles (V)	Rest	5 miles (V)	Rest
WEEK 3	Beginner	4.5 miles (V)	Rest	4.5 miles (V)	Rest	4.5 miles (V)	Rest	5 miles (V)
	Advanced	5.5 miles (V)	Rest	5.5 miles (M)	Rest	5.5 miles (V)	Rest	6 miles (V)
WEEK 4	Beginner	Rest	5 miles (M)	Rest	5 miles (V)	Rest	5.5 miles (V)	Rest
	Advanced	Rest	6 miles (V)	Rest	5 miles (M)	Rest	6 miles (V)	5 miles (I)
WEEK 5	Beginner	4 miles (V)	Rest	4.5 miles (M)	Rest	4.5 miles (V)	Rest	4.5 miles (V)
	Advanced	Rest	6.5 miles (V)	Rest	5 miles (M)	Rest	6 miles (V)	5 miles (I)
WEEK 6	Beginner	Rest	5 miles (I)	Rest	6 miles (V)	Rest	5 miles (M)	6 miles (V)
	Advanced	Rest	7 miles (V)	Rest	5 miles (M)	Rest	6 miles (V)	5 miles (I)
WEEK 7	Beginner	Rest	5 miles (I)	Rest	6 miles (V)	Rest	5 miles (M)	6 miles (V)
	Advanced	Rest	7 miles (M)	Rest	6 miles (V)	Rest	5 miles (I)	6 miles (V)
WEEK 8	Beginner	Rest	5 miles (V)	Rest	4 miles (V)	Rest	Rest	Race
	Advanced	Rest	6 miles (V)	Rest	5 miles (V)	Rest	Rest	Race

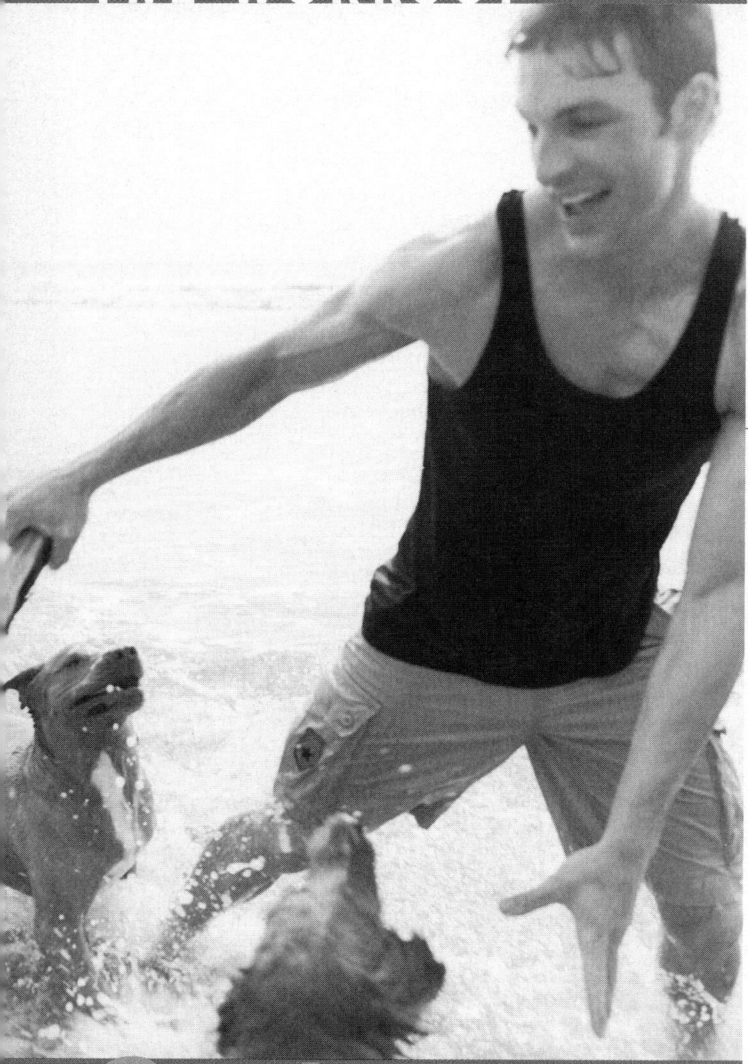

Run faster than ever with our 3-week speed-building program

Whether you're sprinting out of the blocks, stealing second base, or making a fast break for the basket, speed is what you need. And no matter what your sport, this 3-week workout will leave your opponent in the dust. Get ready for takeoff.

Instructions

Choose the beginner workout if you have less than a year of strength-training experience, or if you're coming back from a layoff of longer than 4 months. Choose the intermediate/advanced program if you've been working out consistently for the past year or longer.

If you belong to a gym, you can do the exercises exactly as shown here. Or, if you prefer, you can replace machine exercises with the alternate versions using a barbell or dumbbells. If you work out at home, you can do any of these exercises using a barbell or dumbbells, or you can make use of your multistation home gym.

Sprint Condition

BY MICHAEL MEJIA, C.S.C.S.

Perform the beginner workout 3 days a week, resting a day after each workout. So you might do the workout on Monday, Wednesday, and Friday. Do each pair of exercises as a superset, performing them back-to-back with no rest in between. After each superset, rest 60 seconds, then do the next pair of exercises, until you've completed one set of each exercise in the workout. In other words, you'll perform the entire workout as a modified circuit, completing your first set of each exercise before you start your second set. Do four to six repetitions of the first exercise in each superset (the "explosive lifts") and 10 to 12 repetitions of the second. Complete a total of two circuits in each workout. On one of your "rest" days, do four 40-yard sprints, resting 2 minutes after each. Increase the number of sprints you perform by one or two each week.

SUPERSET 1

BARBELL JUMP SQUAT

● Use a light weight—perhaps one-third of what you'd work with on back squats—and go for speed and power. (Stay away from this one if you've had back problems.) Set your barbell on the squat supports, so you have to bend your knees slightly to step under it and set it on your shoulders. (You don't want to have to lift it up to the supports at the end of a set— you may not be able to reach them.) Position yourself under the bar, so it rests on the backs of your shoulders and your trapezius, not your neck. (When you pull your shoulder blades back, your traps should form a nice shelf for the bar. It shouldn't hurt at all; if it does, it's a sure sign you're doing something wrong.) Hold the bar with a wide, overhand grip, straighten your legs to lift it off the rack, step back, and set your feet shoulder-width apart with your knees slightly bent and your lower back in its naturally arched position. Then squat down quickly until your thighs are at a 45-degree angle with the floor.

● Immediately change directions, and push from your calves to straighten your body so explosively that your feet come off the floor a few inches. Land as softly as possible on your toes, then immediately descend back to the starting position as you shift your weight to your heels.

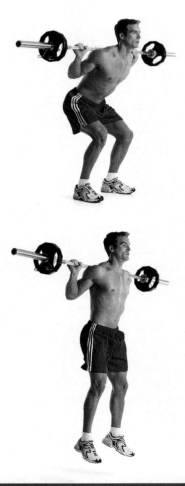

NEUTRAL-GRIP NEGATIVE PULLUP (Alternate: Pullover)

● Set a bench under parallel chinup bars to help you reach the bars. Grasp the parallel bars using an overhand grip, with your palms facing each other. Give yourself a boost from the bench, so you don't have to use much effort to pull your chest up next to your hands. (The work comes in the next part of the move.) Cross your ankles behind you.

● Lower yourself as slowly as you can, then jump up to the starting position and repeat.

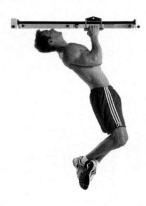

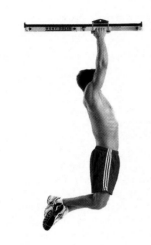

SUPERSET 2

PLYOMETRIC PUSHUP

● On a well-padded carpet or an exercise mat, assume the basic pushup position. Support your body with the balls of your feet and with your hands, positioning the latter slightly wider than shoulder-width apart, palms flat on the floor. Straighten your arms without locking your elbows. Then lower your torso until your chest is just a fraction of an inch off the floor.

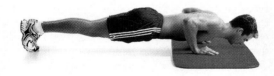

● Quickly push up with enough force so that your hands come off the floor. (You may have seen guys do this with a hand clap. Don't bother—it's just for show, and it increases your injury risk.) Catch yourself with your elbows slightly bent, then lower yourself with a controlled movement.

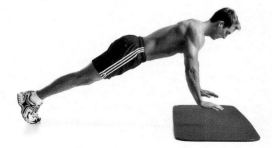

DUMBBELL REVERSE LUNGE

● Stand with two dumbbells hanging at arm's length. Pull your shoulder blades back and your belly in, so your torso stays erect throughout the move.

● Step back 2 to 3 feet (depending on your leg length) with one foot, allowing only the ball of that foot to touch the floor behind you. As you step (not after), lower the knee of your receding leg to 2 or 3 inches above the floor. Your front leg should end up bent about 90 degrees, with that knee over the toes. Quickly switch direction, and push yourself back up.

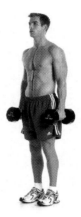
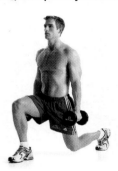

SUPERSET 3

BARBELL POWER CLEAN

● Squat over a loaded barbell on the floor, and grip it overhand at shoulder width—just as if you were starting a standard deadlift.

● Pull the bar off the floor as fast as you can, go up on your toes, shrug your shoulders, and perform an upright row as you lift the bar up along your body.

● When the bar hits chest level, "catch" it on your front shoulders by dropping under it in a half-squat and turning your palms up toward the ceiling. Your upper arms should be parallel to the floor when the bar lands on your shoulders. Stand up straight, then lower the bar to the floor and return to the starting position.

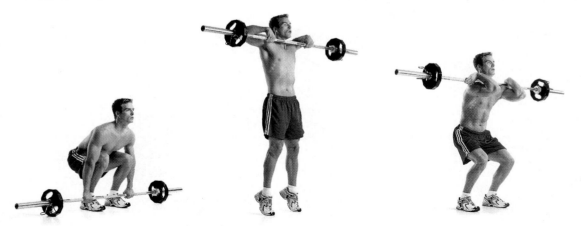

CABLE SEATED ROW (Alternate: Bent-Over Row)

● Attach a short straight bar to the low pulley, and set a pair of 45-pound weight plates on the floor to either side of the pulley. Grab the bar with a false (thumbs on the same side as the fingers), overhand, shoulder-width grip. Sit on the floor about 2½ feet in front of the low pulley, with your arms straight, your feet braced against the weight plates, and your torso erect.

● Start the movement by pinching your shoulder blades together in back, then pull the bar to the lower part of your sternum. Keep your elbows up. Pause, then slowly return to the starting position.

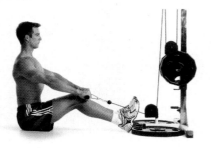
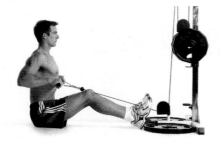

SUPERSET 4

LUNGE JUMP

● Keeping your torso erect, stand with one foot 2 feet ahead of you and the other 2 feet behind and your toes pointed forward. Your front foot should be flat on the floor, but only the ball of your back foot should be planted. To help keep yourself balanced, line up each foot with its corresponding buttock, not with the other foot. Bend both knees to lower your body straight down until your front thigh is halfway to parallel to the floor.

● Then quickly switch directions, and push yourself back up with enough force to propel your entire body off the floor. While in the air, scissor-kick your legs so you land with the opposite leg forward.

● As soon as you land, lower yourself and jump into the next rep. Don't pause between reps—pop them off as fast as you can without sacrificing good form.

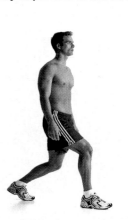
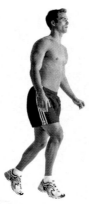
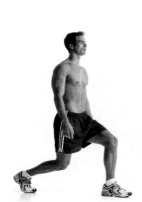

SITUP

● Lie on an exercise mat with your knees bent and your feet together and flat on the floor.

● Holding your hands behind your ears, slowly lift your upper body by using your abs to flex your spine, bringing your chest toward your knees. Roll back down, slowly and with control.

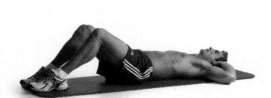 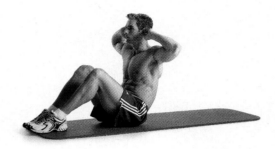

SUPERSET 5

BARBELL PUSH PRESS

● Rest the loaded barbell on the fronts of your shoulders, keeping your elbows in close to your body. Bend your knees, and lower yourself to a half-squat position.

● Immediately drive yourself up with your legs as you thrust the weight toward the ceiling until you are up on your toes and your arms are straightened above you. Slowly return to the starting position.

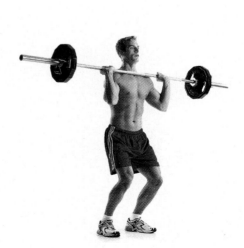 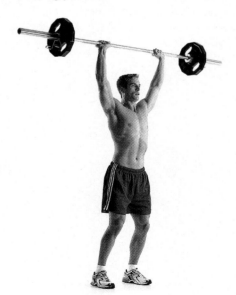

RUSSIAN TWIST

● Start with your torso at a 45- to 60-degree angle to the floor (as if you were halfway through a situp) and your arms raised directly out in front of you. Bend your knees and keep your feet free, not anchored by anything.

● While maintaining this torso angle, rotate as far as possible to one side and then, without pausing, to the other.

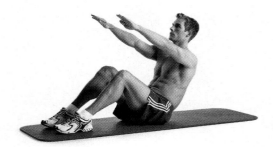 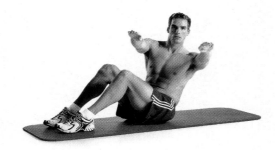

SUPERSET 6

MEDICINE BALL SIDE THROW

● You need a medicine ball and a solid surface, such as a brick or concrete wall, to throw against. (Your living room wall won't cut it—that is, unless you want a gaping hole in the drywall.) Stand about 3 feet from the wall with your feet shoulder-width apart. The wall should be to your left as you hold the ball on your right side.

● Swing it a bit farther to the right, then quickly switch directions and throw it, as hard as you can, to your left, aiming for the wall. You could also do this exercise with a partner to catch the ball and throw it back to you.

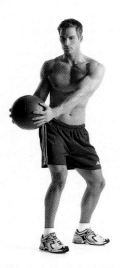 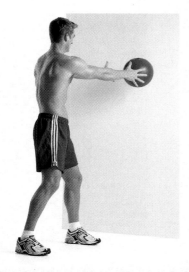

DUMBBELL SINGLE-LEG STANDING CALF RAISE

● Grab a dumbbell in your nondominant hand, and stand on the ball of that foot on a step or wooden block. Rest the instep of your other foot across the Achilles tendon of your working ankle. Hold onto something sturdy with your free hand if you need to. Lower your working heel off the edge of the step as far as your calf will stretch.

● Push your working heel straight up as high as you can. Pause, then return to the starting position. Finish the set with that leg, then repeat with the other.

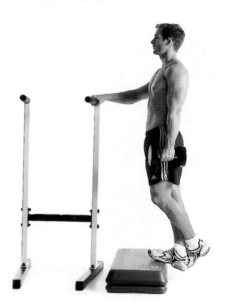

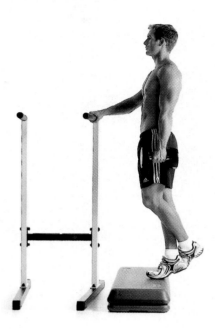

Perform the intermediate/advanced workout 3 days a week, resting a day after each workout. So you might do the workout on Monday, Wednesday, and Friday. Do each pair of exercises as a superset, performing them back-to-back with no rest in between. After each superset, rest 60 seconds, then do the next pair of exercises, until you've completed one set of each exercise in the workout. In other words, you'll perform the entire workout as a modified circuit, completing your first set of each exercise before you start your second set. Do three to five repetitions of the first exercise in each superset (the "explosive lifts") and 6 to 10 repetitions of the second exercise in each superset. Complete a total of two circuits in each workout. On 1 or 2 of your "rest" days, do six 40-yard sprints, resting 2 minutes between sprints. Increase the number of sprints you perform by one or two each week.

SUPERSET 1

BARBELL JUMP SQUAT

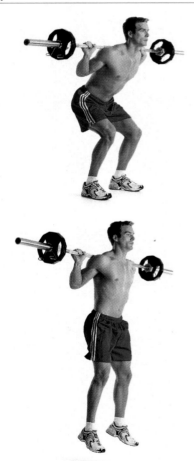

● Use a light weight—perhaps one-third of what you'd work with on back squats—and go for speed and power. (Stay away from this one if you've had back problems.) Set your barbell on the squat supports, so you have to bend your knees slightly to step under it and set it on your shoulders. (You don't want to have to lift it up to the supports at the end of a set—you may not be able to reach them.) Position yourself under the bar, so it rests on the backs of your shoulders and your trapezius, not your neck. (When you pull your shoulder blades back, your traps should form a nice shelf for the bar. It shouldn't hurt at all; if it does, it's a sure sign you're doing something wrong.) Hold the bar with a wide, overhand grip, straighten your legs to lift it off the rack, step back, and set your feet shoulder-width apart with your knees slightly bent and your lower back in its naturally arched position. Then squat down quickly until your thighs are at a 45-degree angle with the floor.

● Immediately change directions, and push from your calves to straighten your body so explosively that your feet come off the floor a few inches. Land as softly as possible on your toes, then immediately descend back to the starting position as you shift your weight to your heels.

BARBELL SQUAT

● Set your barbell on the squat supports, so you have to bend your knees slightly to step under it and set it on your shoulders. (You don't want to have to lift it up to the supports at the end of a set—you may not be able to reach them.) Position yourself under the bar so it rests on the backs of your shoulders and your trapezius, not your neck. (When you pull your shoulder blades back, your traps should form a nice shelf for the bar. It shouldn't hurt at all; if it does, it's a sure sign you're doing something wrong.) Hold the bar with a wide, overhand grip, straighten your legs to lift it off the rack, step back, and set your feet shoulder-width apart with your knees slightly bent and your lower back in its naturally arched position.

● Initiating the descent at the hips, not the knees, lower yourself as though sitting in a chair behind you. Stop when the tops of your thighs are parallel to the floor, pause, then push back up to the starting position. Your knees should stay in line with your feet throughout the movement; they shouldn't splay out or pinch in.

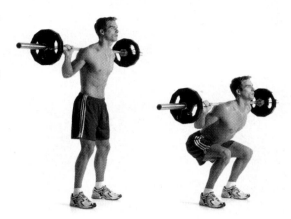

SUPERSET 2

BARBELL POWER CLEAN

● Squat over a loaded barbell on the floor, and grip it overhand at shoulder width—just as if you were starting a standard deadlift.

● Pull the bar off the floor as fast as you can, go up on your toes, shrug your shoulders, and perform an upright row as you lift the bar up along your body.

● When the bar hits chest level, "catch" it on your front shoulders by dropping under it in a half-squat and turning your palms up toward the ceiling. Your upper arms should be parallel to the floor when the bar lands on your shoulders. Stand up straight, then lower the bar to the floor and return to the starting position.

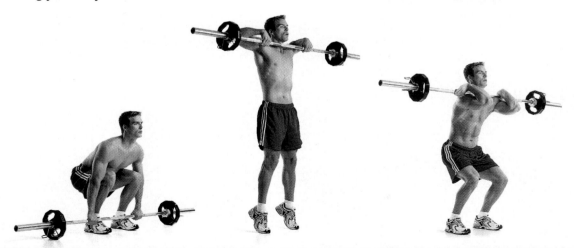

CABLE SEATED ROW (Alternate: Bent-Over Row)

● Attach a short straight bar to the low pulley, and set a pair of 45-pound weight plates on the floor to either side of the pulley. Grab the bar with a false (thumbs on the same side as the fingers), overhand, shoulder-width grip. Sit on the floor about 2½ feet in front of the low pulley, with your arms straight, your feet braced against the weight plates, and your torso erect.

● Start the movement by pinching your shoulder blades together in back, then pull the bar to the lower part of your sternum. Keep your elbows up. Pause, then slowly return to the starting position.

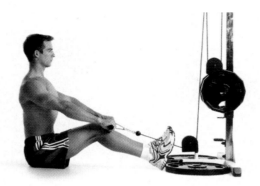 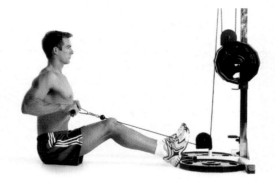

SUPERSET 3

PLYOMETRIC PUSHUP

● On a well-padded carpet or an exercise mat, assume the basic pushup position. Support your body with the balls of your feet and with your hands, positioning the latter slightly wider than shoulder-width apart, palms flat on the floor. Straighten your arms without locking your elbows. Then lower your torso until your chest is just a fraction of an inch off the floor.

● Quickly push up with enough force so that your hands come off the floor. (You may have seen guys do this with a hand clap. Don't bother—it's just for show, and it increases your injury risk.) Catch yourself with your elbows slightly bent, then lower yourself with a controlled movement.

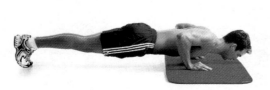 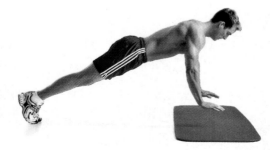

DUMBBELL BENCH PRESS

● Lie on a flat bench holding two dumbbells over your middle chest with an overhand grip and straight arms.

● Pinching your shoulder blades back, bend your elbows and slowly lower the dumbbells until they're right next to your armpits, a few inches higher than chest level. Pause, then press the dumbbells back up, bringing your hands close together without clanking the weights.

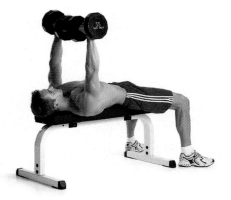

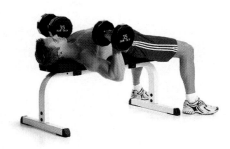

SUPERSET 4

MEDICINE BALL SIDE THROW

● You need a medicine ball and a solid surface, such as a brick or concrete wall, to throw against. (Your living room wall won't cut it—that is, unless you want a gaping hole in the drywall.) Stand about 3 feet from the wall with your feet shoulder-width apart. The wall should be to your left as you hold the ball on your right side.

● Swing it a bit farther to the right, then quickly switch directions and throw it, as hard as you can, to your left, aiming for the wall. You could also do this exercise with a partner to catch the ball and throw it back to you.

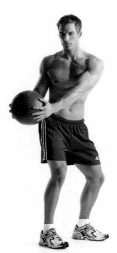

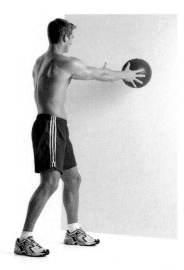

WEIGHTED RUSSIAN TWIST

● Sitting on the floor with your knees bent and your feet flat, hold a light weight plate with your arms extended straight out in front of you. Lean back until your torso is at a 60- to 75-degree angle from the floor. Pull your belly in.

● Twist your torso as far as you can to one side and then to the other to complete the rep.

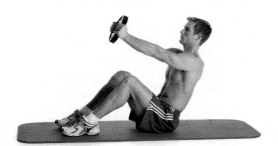
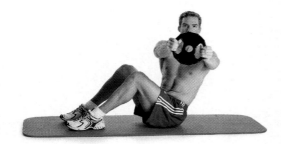

SUPERSET 5

DUMBBELL LUNGE JUMP

● Holding a pair of dumbbells at arm's length, stand with your torso erect and with one foot 2 feet ahead of you and the other 2 feet behind, toes pointed forward. Your front foot should be flat on the floor, but only the ball of your back foot should be planted. To help keep yourself balanced, line up each foot with its corresponding buttock, not with the other foot. Bend both knees to lower your body straight down until your front thigh is not quite parallel to the floor.

● Then quickly switch directions, and push yourself back up with enough force to propel your entire body off the floor. While in the air, scissor-kick your legs so you land with the opposite leg forward.

● As soon as you land, lower yourself and jump into the next rep. Don't pause between reps—pop them off as fast as you can without sacrificing good form.

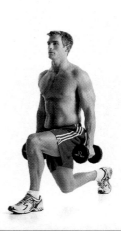
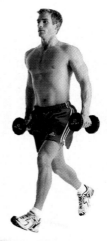
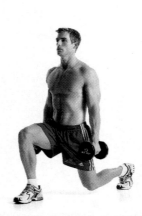

V-UP

● Lie on an exercise mat with your legs straight out on the floor and your arms straight up in the air, fingers pointing toward the ceiling.

● Contracting your abs, fold your body up by lifting your legs off the floor and stretching your arms toward your toes. Keep your back straight. Pause at your full extension, then return to the starting position.

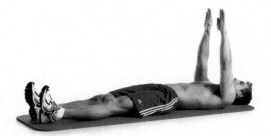
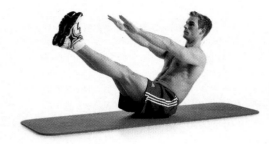

WEIGHTED SITUP

● Lie on an exercise mat in the situp position—knees bent, feet flat on the floor. With both hands, hold the ends of a dumbbell in your upper chest, just below your chin.

● Slowly lift your upper body by using your abs to flex your spine, bringing your chest toward your knees. Roll back down, slowly and with control.

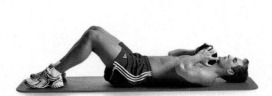
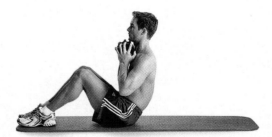

This workout series is adapted from *The Men's Health Home Workout Bible*, by Lou Schuler, with exercise programs by Michael Mejia, M.S., C.S.C.S. © 2002 by Rodale Inc. Available wherever books are sold.

TRAINING TIPS

Q **Every runner I know has hamstring problems. How can I avoid them?**

A.B., LANDOVER, MARYLAND

A If you have weak or tight hamstrings, your body may compensate by tilting your pelvis forward, placing stress on your lower back. Next stop: injury and postural abnormalities. To build hamstrings that will fight all that, try the Swiss ball curl, advises Robert dos Remedios, C.S.C.S., director of speed, strength, and conditioning at the College of

GET IT RIGHT

Hamstring Stretch

Stand up and put your left heel on a chair to stretch your left hamstring. Bend at the hips until you feel the stretch. Now look down at your right foot. Where is it pointing?

"No one puts his foot in the correct position, which is pointing forward," says Bill Bandy, Ph.D., a professor of physical therapy at the University of Central Arkansas. "When the foot points to the side, you're working the groin, not the hamstrings." Feel the difference?

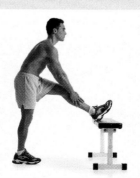

the Canyons in Santa Clarita, California. The instability of the ball will train you well for jarring sports, bumpy roads, and the current job market. Here's how to do the ball curl: Lie on the floor with your calves on top of a Swiss ball, your upper back and shoulders on the floor, and your arms out to the sides. Raise your hips and your lower back off the ground, so they form a straight line with your legs.

Keeping your abs tight, pull the ball toward your butt by digging your heels into the ball until your feet are flat and your knees and butt are high in the air.

Pause, then push the ball away from you until your legs are straight. Do 5 to 10 repetitions. When this gets too easy, double the resistance by lifting one leg off the ball and pulling the ball with your other leg.

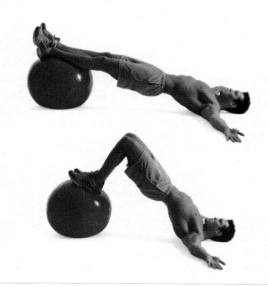

Avoid the Sand Trap

Headed for a beach vacation? You'd be wise to skip the beach run you've been day-dreaming about. While you may think running on the beach is good for your feet and legs, it's not. Sand is too soft and uneven, placing extra strain on the ankle and foot ligaments, which can lead to ankle sprains, stress fractures, and bone bruising, says Timothy Downs, D.P.M., a podiatrist in Chelmsford, Massachusetts. If you can't resist that bikini-ogling beach jog, wear shoes and run on the harder, wet sand.

FRIGID AIR

Cold air makes my ears and lungs ache when I run outside. Should I worry?

T.G., ASHEVILLE, NORTH CAROLINA

Not at all. But you might try breathing through both your mouth and nose to help warm the air before it reaches your lungs. If your inner ear hurts, you may have an infection. Or the temperature difference between the outside air and your inner ear could be to blame. Get a doctor to rule out an infection, then wear a knit cap.

BURNING QUESTION

My left Achilles tendon burns at the start of a run. The pain goes away after I cool down. Is my tendon about to snap?

V.P., DOTHAN, ALABAMA

Not if you heed the warning signs of Achilles tendinitis. Your tendon probably has some tears, which are causing inflammation and pain and could lead to a rupture. So warm up slowly, stretching well: Lean against a wall with both hands, put one foot flat on the ground and slightly forward, and place the other flat on the ground behind you. Press against the wall, and feel the stretch in the back of your leg. Do this for 3 to 4 minutes. Believe us, this extra time is much less aggravation than months on crutches—which is exactly what you're facing if the tendon ruptures. If warming up doesn't eliminate the pain, check with a trainer or doctor about your running technique and shoes. Either one could be the source of the problem.

GIVE 110 PERCENT?

I've been using a heart monitor to exercise at 60 percent of my maximum heart rate (MHR). What would happen if I exercised at 110 percent?

E.R., BURLINGTON, VERMONT

You can't. MHR is an absolute limit. You might not think so, though, because the heart rate formula—220 beats per minute, minus your age—has a 10 percent margin of error, according to Richard Stein, M.D., a spokesman for the American Heart Association. The only sure way to pin down the number is to have your doctor administer a treadmill test to exhaustion, says Stein. Once you know your max, you should train at 60 to 80 percent of it. You'll see a modest effect on your fitness level at 60 and a good effect at 80, but beyond that, you're wasting effort.

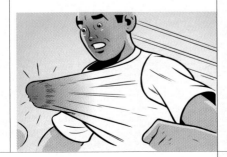

BLACK OUT

I've been running more, and now one of my toenails is turning black. What do I do?

S.L., DENTON, TEXAS

First, lose your sneaks. They don't fit right, and your toe is sliding into the toebox, causing bleeding under the nail. A half size smaller—or a different model—should work better.

"Black toe" looks ugly, but the bleeding will stop. The nail may survive, or it could eventually fall off. If it really hurts, get a doctor to pierce it to relieve the pressure. Lay off the running until the pain goes away.

RUBBER NECKING

My neck hurts when I run on a treadmill. The pain extends down into my shoulder blade. What am I doing wrong?

M.P., LOVELAND, COLORADO

First, quit swiveling to check out the chicks in spandex. Second, take a look at your running mechanics. Sometimes people tense their shoulders and trapezius muscles when running. Stretch your neck before, during, and after the workout. And every 5 minutes or so, let your arms dangle by your sides for 15 seconds to relax your upper body. There could be a neurological cause for your pain. It's possible that a nerve is pinched or irritated. If you experience tingling or numbness in your shoulders or down your arms, see a neurologist or rehabilitation specialist.

KNEE SAVER

I run 5 miles a day, and my knees cause me trouble. Can SAM-e stop the pain?

P.B., SEATTLE

Assuming you don't just need new shoes, this supplement may work. SAM-e is an amino acid believed to help with joint pain and cartilage repair. (Just stay away from it if you have a history of

HEAL YOURSELF

Save Your Soles

Sharp heel and arch pain when your feet hit the floor in the morning either means you stepped on the remote, or you're suffering from plantar fasciitis. It's a common inflammation of the tissue on the underside of your foot. These stretches can help you hit the ground running.

While still in bed. "After any prolonged period of rest, the plantar fascia ligament tightens and is susceptible to tearing when you step down," says Timothy Downs, D.P.M. Before leaving horizontal, cross the leg of your injured foot (let's say your right) over your left leg. Pull the toes toward your right shin. Hold for 10 seconds, rest, and repeat nine times.

After getting up. Lean against a wall, put the aching foot in front of the other, and point the toes of your back foot toward the heel of

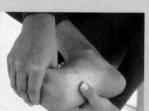

your front foot. Your back leg should be straight and your front knee bent. Hold for 10 seconds, and repeat nine times.

During the day. While sitting, roll a bottle under the arch of your foot to keep your ligaments loose.

manic depression.) The usual dose is 400 milligrams (mg) a day, but start with 200 mg, before meals, at first. You should start taking B_6, B_{12}, and folic acid to avoid a buildup of homocysteine.

SECRETS TO SUCCESS

Why do Kenyans win so many marathons—and how can I tap their secrets for my next 10-K?

J.Y., ATLANTA

Lots of reasons, including practice, practice, practice. They're training at world-class levels, after all. Many experts also argue genetics, in which case you're either Kenyan or you're not. Some research boils it down to speed training and max VO_2 (the volume of oxygen you can consume while exercising at maximum capacity)—things you can improve. One study found that Kenyan runners can run at 94 percent of their peak velocity for 10 kilometers, and other studies have determined that their max VO_2 is consistently higher than that of any other group. Genetics? Maybe. But one researcher suspects that their speed and max VO_2

can be attributed to the recruitment of more muscle fibers in their legs.

For you, that means hills. Lots of hills. Running uphill increases oxygen consumption, while running downhill builds the leg muscles through "eccentric contractions," when the muscle is extended, says Amby Burfoot, executive editor of *Runner's World*. That makes for stronger muscles and more resistance to fatigue and soreness, "which can translate into speed," says Burfoot.

Another Kenyan trick: They're skinny. Burfoot estimates that every pound of excess weight on your frame adds 2 seconds to your mile time. Lose 10 pounds of fat, shave 20 seconds off your mile pace. Try tempo running, too: Run for 20 minutes at 90 percent of your maximum heart rate as part of your training program once a week or once every 2 weeks, depending on your level of fitness. (World-class Kenyan runners can do this for up to 70 minutes.)

WAKE-UP CALL

Why do some of my toes go to sleep when I run?

J.W., BURLINGTON, VERMONT

EAT AND RUN

Don't Forgo Fat

A low-fat diet may increase your risk of injuries from running, a new University of Buffalo study reports. Researchers tracked 87 runners for a year and found that those who got fewer than 30 percent of their calories a day from fat were also the most likely to incur running-related injuries. The study's authors believe diets low in fat may limit the amount of nutrients available to repair muscle damage after a run.

Your problem is almost certainly running shoes that are too small or tied too tightly. The wrong fit can cause numbness—the nerves in your foot are compressed, or bloodflow is restricted. There's a slim chance the problem could be peripheral neuropathy (damaged nerves in your extremities) or arterial insufficiency (poor blood supply). Change your gear, socks included. If the numbness doesn't go away in a couple of weeks, have your doctor test for a bigger problem.

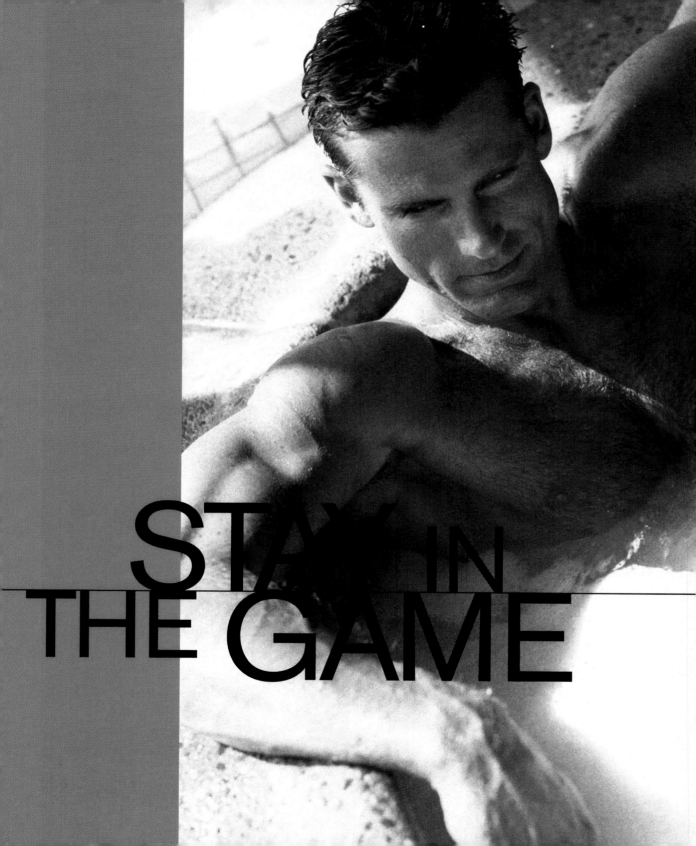

STAY IN THE GAME

Guys and sports are inseparable. We're like peanut butter and jelly, beer and chips. No matter what our age, the playing field calls to us. Be it a game of hoops, a round of 18, or nine innings of ball, we live for the game. Which is why being sidelined with an injury can be so frustrating, not to mention painful.

As with anything else, the best sports medicine is prevention. Learn ways to increase flexibility and correct muscle imbalances that often lead to injuries—to keep you healthy all season long. But of course, especially in contact sports, the errant elbow to the jaw or line drive to the head happens. To make sure the game goes on, learn on-the-spot strategies for treating common sports injuries, plus how to know when to let the ER doc take care of it for you.

If signs of aging are slowing you down—joint pain or muscle aches—we've got remedies for those, too: workouts and supplements that are proven to do the trick.

While staying injury-free is important, living until your next match or workout is a whole different ball game. It's the scary irony of fitness. Some guys who are ultrafit just drop dead in mid-stride. At ripe old ages of 51, 52. Find out why and what warning signs to look out for, so you'll be alive and well . . . while your opponent? We hope you knock 'em dead.

BY LOU SCHULER

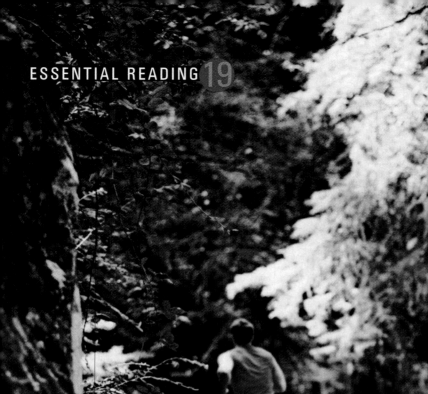

Dying to Be Fit

Hundreds of guys—including some of the world's fittest men—have taken their final breaths while exercising. Here's how to make it to your next workout

G uy goes out for a run. It's just a 4-miler—nothing, really, to a seasoned marathoner who usually runs 10 miles a day, 7 days a week. Nobody knows why he stops 40 or 50 yards short of his front door—maybe he's checking his pulse, maybe he's tying a shoe—but everybody knows what happens next to Jim Fixx, the 52-year-old patron saint of running: He dies.

You've probably heard that story. But you may not know about Edmund Burke, Ph.D., who was to serious endurance cycling what Fixx was to running. He died on a training ride last fall, at age 53.

And you almost certainly haven't heard of Frederick Montz, David Nagey, or Jeffrey Williams, three brilliant physicians at Johns Hopkins University who died while running. The oldest of the three was 51.

You'd think that exercise icons should live to be 100. And yet, every year, a few of them go permanently offline at half that age.

Two questions arise. The first is obvious: Why do the hearts of such highly conditioned men fail during exercise designed to make their hearts stronger? The second is so radical it borders on treason against the health and fitness cause: Is there something wrong with the entire notion of endurance exercise as a healthy, life-extending activity?

I've been skeptical about the benefits of aerobic exercise for years. But the answers surprised even me. Pull up a chair—you'll want to be sitting down when you read this.

PEAK performance

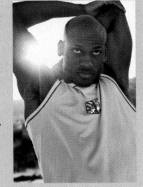

Stretch Your Limits

A new U.S. government–funded study by the National Institutes of Health shows that stretching and strength training twice a week may help reduce the risk of exercise-related injury by about 45 percent in men, according to Jennifer Hootman, Ph.D., an epidemiologist at the Centers for Disease Control and Prevention.

The type of stretching you do probably doesn't matter much. Another recent study, this one at the Medical College of Ohio in Toledo, shows that the total time you spend stretching matters more than the amount of time you hold any single stretch.

The Road to Nowhere

The idea that a well-trained endurance athlete could just drop dead was unfathomable a generation ago. Thomas Bassler, M.D., went so far as to say that anyone who could finish a marathon in less than 4 hours could not have serious heart problems. He conducted a study on 14 marathoners who had died of cardiovascular disease, and concluded that all were malnourished. Unfortunately, he reported this conclusion in the July 27, 1984, edition of the *Journal of the American Medical Association*. Fixx had died 7 days earlier.

Nobody today believes that endurance training confers immunity to anything, whether it's sudden death from heart disease or the heartbreak of psoriasis. Every time you lace up your running shoes, there's a chance your final kick will involve a bucket, and every expert knows this.

"I think the risk is inescapable, and it's bigger than we're letting on," says Paul Thompson, M.D., director of preventive cardiology at Hartford Hospital in Connecticut and a researcher who studies sudden death and exercise. One of Thompson's studies showed that 10 percent of the heart attacks treated at his hospital were exercise related.

Exercise Caution

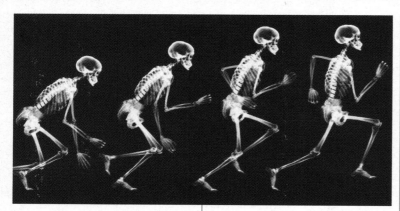

You're young and you're extremely fit. Almost always, that's a good thing. But in rare cases, a high fitness level hides—and may even help cause—a heart disorder known as ARVD. It's a genetic condition in which the muscle of the right ventricle turns into fatty or fibrous tissue.

Signs of ARVD (arrhythmogenic right-ventricular dysplasia) and other stealthy cardiac disorders include the following:

- Passing out, especially during exercise
- Heart palpitations, especially during exercise

- Sudden death of a family member, particularly a sibling or parent, before age 60

A heart attack "out of the blue" might be an indication of a hidden genetic condition.

In ARVD, as the right ventricular muscle changes, abnormal heart rhythms occur, leading to the symptoms. If you're worried, go to a doctor—a series of noninvasive tests can determine whether you have the disorder. The Web site arvd.com can give you more information.

Ironically, patients with

ARVD can be very fit athletes; extreme exercise may trigger the condition in those with the inherited susceptibility, says Hugh Calkins, M.D., director of electrophysiology at the Johns Hopkins Hospital. Moreover, young, athletic men often shrug off the warning signs.

ARVD affects about 1 in 5,000 people but may be the cause of up to 20 percent of sudden cardiac deaths in people under the age of 35.

Coronary artery disease and heart attacks account for about 80 percent of the sudden cardiac deaths in America each year. ARVD and other inherited conditions cause the rest, Calkins says. These disorders, which affect men more than women, include long QT syndrome and Brugada syndrome (problems with electrical impulses in the heart) and hypertrophic cardiomyopathy (thickening of the heart muscle).

"Those heart attacks tend to be in people who aren't fit," he says. "But that doesn't mean that's the only group that gets it, unfortunately. There are these very fit guys who go out for a run and drop dead."

Thompson's studies and others show that the chances of sudden death are about one in every 15,000 to 18,000 exercisers per year. That comes to one death for every 1.5 million exercise bouts. Curiously, the most serious endurance athletes seem to be at the greatest risk. Here's how it breaks down, according to an often-cited 1982 study published in the *New England Journal of Medicine*:

- One death per 17,000 men who exercise vigorously 1 to 19 minutes a week

- One death per 23,000 men who exercise vigorously 20 to 139 minutes a week

- One death per 13,000 men who exercise vigorously 140 or more minutes a week

I had to look at the chart twice to see its startling conclusion: The highest death rate is among the men who exercise long and hard, and it's much higher than that of the men who exercise short and hard. Worse, the guys who do hardly any vigorous exercise had a lower death rate than the guys who do the most.

About a zillion studies—I lost count in the millions—have shown that aerobic exercise leads to a healthier heart and a longer life.

So I have to wonder why more of such a healthy activity is worse, rather than better.

Sweatin' to the Oldies

In 1970, a study of San Francisco longshoremen made a strong argument that physical activity helps prevent heart disease. The longshoremen who got promoted to mostly sedentary management positions developed heart disease 25 percent more often than those who worked on their feet. An important note about this study and similar ones that preceded it: The subjects weren't doing formal, steady-pace endurance exercise. They were walking and stopping, lifting things up and putting them down. Numerous formal exercise studies followed, many of them attempting to quantify how

(continued on page 176)

PAINkiller

Rub It In
Do Icy Hot and Bengay really work on sore muscles?

N.P., Hagerstown, Maryland

Some people swear by these topical pain relievers. The active ingredients are usually menthol, to send blood rushing to the area—which creates the burning sensation and can help healing—and camphor to cool the skin. But these creams treat the symptoms, not the cause. Massage and stretching will do a lot more for your sore muscles—without leaving a nauseating vapor trail.

The Easiest Hard Workout in the World

If you can spare 60 minutes a month, you just might save your life

BY LOU SCHULER

The LifeWaves program is simple: Work like hell for 45 seconds, then sit on your butt until your heart rate returns to its pre-exertion level. Work, rest, repeat. It was created by Irv Dardik, M.D., based on the premise that exercise should include both stress and recovery. Many of us are good at the stress part of it, working our heart rates up, but almost nobody trains his heart rate to fall. And yet it's during the fall that the best-trained athletes are the most vulnerable. Some of these guys are so fit and have such low resting heart rates that a quick drop can turn into a cardiac tailspin from which the exerciser never recovers. Result: death by exercise, or, more accurately, death by lack of recovery from exercise.

So Dardik's LifeWaves program teaches your heart rate to go up—way up—in a short but intense effort. Then you sit down and teach your heart to slow down rapidly but safely in the next 2 to 5 minutes. You start the next cycle when you've fully recovered from the previous one.

A workout typically involves five or six of these cycles. By the last cycle, you should reach your maximum heart rate. An average program might involve 60 minutes of exercise— a month.

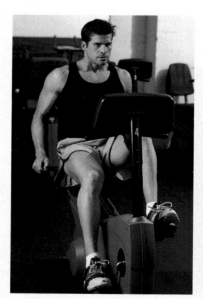

Heart rate: 72, rising to 163

Step 1 Strap on a heart-rate monitor and pump away for 45 seconds, driving your heart rate up.

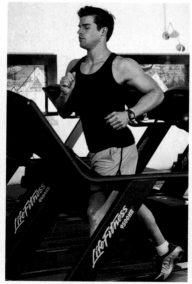

Heart rate: 170, falling to 89

Step 2 Rest until your heart rate approaches its pre-exercise rate—between 2 and 5 minutes— then repeat.

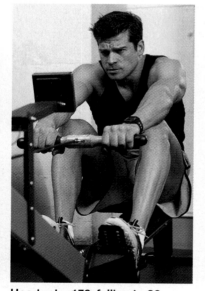

Heart rate: 170, falling to 89

Step 3 Continue the routine on the same or different equipment, again letting your heart rate drop afterward.

I wouldn't have heard of Irv Dardik if he didn't have a book deal and other business partnerships with Rodale, the company that owns *Men's Health*. But as soon as a coworker described his ideas to me, I knew I had to meet him and try his workout.

Dardik, who's 66, tells me he can bring his heart rate up to 190 beats per minute. If you use the standard equation for predicting maximum heart rate—220 minus your age—his max should be 154. A major

part of his LifeWaves theory is that you should strive to maintain a wide margin between your maximum and minimum heart rates throughout life, rather than settle for a slow decline in the range. Decline is death. A 2002 study in the *New England Journal of Medicine* showed this convincingly: Researchers tracked 6,213 men who had been told they needed to exercise for various reasons. Those who died in the 6 years of the study had the lowest

maximal heart rates and the lowest exercise capacity.

I can't tell you if the Life-Waves workout will save any lives. I think it will, but it's a nearly impossible theory to prove. If nothing else, Dardik's program could appeal to the majority of Americans who don't exercise at all, since 60 minutes of exertion a month sounds a lot easier then the official recommendation of 30 minutes a day.

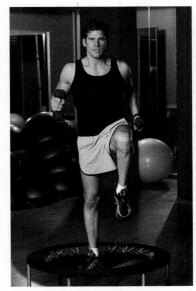

Heart rate: 170, falling to 94

Step 4 By the fourth cycle, your heart won't make it all the way back to its pre-exercise rate. That's okay.

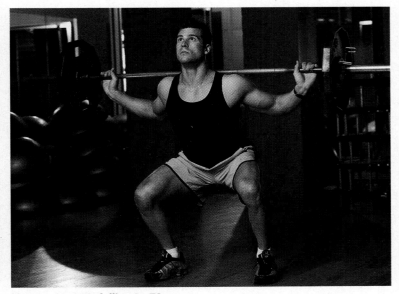

Heart rate: 190, falling to 72

Step 5 After four or five cycles, it's time for the final wave, where you want to get your heart rate up to its max rate (figure 220 beats per minute minus your age). Afterward, give your heart plenty of time to drop to resting speed.

The Best Heart-Rate Monitors

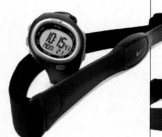

Nike Triax c8

Easy-to-read numbers; most user-friendly of all. ($120; niketown.com)

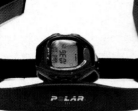

Polar S120

Alarm signals when you miss target heart rate range. ($100; polarusa.com)

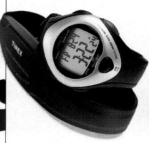

Timex Marathon

Digital FM signal prevents interference from power lines. ($60; timex.com)

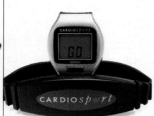

Cardiosport Go

Simple, dependable, no-frills monitor. ($54; strikeitfit.com)

much physical activity is needed to prevent heart disease, and at what intensity levels. The Harvard Alumni Health Study found that heart disease risk starts going down when you expend more than 500 calories a week and continues to decrease until you get to 2,000 calories a week. Then things level off—more exercise doesn't offer more protection.

The bottom number isn't much exercise; a 200-pound man walking 2 hours a week at 3 mph will burn 600 calories. And the top number isn't particularly intimidating, either. Our 200-pounder would have to run about $16^{1}/_{2}$ miles at a 12-minute-mile pace to burn 2,000 calories a week. (Lighter guys will burn fewer calories per minute or mile; bigger men will burn more.)

Intensity is a separate issue, with some studies showing that moderate-intensity ex-

ercise (walking, bowling, playing golf) helps your heart, and others showing little benefit until you start cranking (running, lifting serious iron, playing basketball or soccer).

Still other studies measure heart disease risk by activity level, and these show something really interesting: Once you get past the 75th percentile of physical activity— guys who exercise more than three-quarters of the population—protection against heart disease levels off. In fact, among the most active, it actually declines slightly, according to a review in *Medicine & Science in Sports & Exercise*. In other words, the superactive are more likely to die than the merely active.

Snow Problem

One reason it's so hard to understand the whole death-by-exercise phenomenon is that so few people die during formal exercise—

there are only about 100 cases per year. So it helps to look at those who suffer heart attacks during heavy physical exertion in general, rather than fitness activities in particular. One important study, published in the *New England Journal of Medicine* in 1993, looked at 1,228 nonfatal heart attacks, 54 of which occurred during or soon after serious exertion. (The cutoff point was 6 metabolic units, or METs. This means the exertion was greater than or equal to six times the energy required by a body at rest. Heavy strength training is considered a 6-MET activity, as are wood chopping and snow shoveling; running 12-minute miles racks up 8 METs.)

The researchers divided the cases into three categories and found that about 18 percent of the exercise-induced heart attacks occurred during lifting and pushing, 30 percent during jogging or sports (racquet sports in particular), and 52 percent during yard work, such as splitting wood.

And that brings us to a major cause of death by exertion: snow shoveling.

A researcher at William Beaumont Hospital in Royal Oak, Michigan, tallied 36 snow-related deaths in the Detroit area following two heavy storms. (Curiously, several of the victims were using snowblowers.)

It's easy to see why frozen precipitation scores such a high body count. "Heart rates go up like a maximal treadmill test," says Barry Franklin, Ph.D., director of cardiac rehabilitation and exercise laboratories at the Beaumont hospital. "Combine that with cold weather, which constricts arteries, and you have a prescription for disaster."

An interesting point: The men who shovel off to meet their makers following a snowstorm, or who have to call an EMT after putting ax to wood, aren't doing aerobic activities. There's no endurance component. Snow shoveling and wood chopping are anaerobic activities—strenuous efforts that can't be continued longer than a few minutes without stopping to rest.

In other words, these activities resemble strength training and are very different from running or cycling. So you'd probably guess that weight lifting also has a pumped-up body count.

Nope. In fact, it has virtually no body count. A few guys a year die from dropping barbells on their tracheas, and some strokes turn up in the literature, but you'd be hard-pressed to find any cases of heart attacks associated with weight lifting. Post-cardiac-arrest patients are regularly trained back to health with weights, and I couldn't find any references to any of them dying, either.

Strength training protects your heart in two ways: First, says Franklin, you get a

PAINkiller

Sorry, Charley
Why do I get awful charley horses in the middle of the night, and how can I stop them?

M.S., Eastlake, Ohio

Charley horses can be caused by overexertion, dehydration, and low levels of minerals (magnesium, potassium, calcium, and sodium). Before going to bed, try drinking plenty of water or a glass of juice, stretching, and applying heat. If charley visits again, see a doctor—the pain can also be caused by pinched nerves or poor bloodflow.

predictable increase in diastolic blood pressure, which governs the return of blood to your coronary arteries. (If your blood pressure is 120 over 80, 80 is the diastolic number.) That's different from aerobic exercise, in which systolic blood pressure (the first number) rises but diastolic pressure stays the same or possibly even decreases. Both numbers go up by quite a bit when you lift, which means blood is being pushed back to your heart with equivalent force.

Second, most of us tend to hold our breath briefly while lifting. This increases blood pressure dramatically and used to scare the daylights out of doctors, who feared aneurysms could result. But new research from the University of Alberta in Edmonton shows that brief breath-holding actually exerts a sort of counterpressure on arterial walls that neutralizes the rise in blood pressure. Aneurysm avoided.

In other words, your body seems designed to protect itself during brief, heavy exertion, and lifters shouldn't ever have to worry about death by exercise.

PAINkiller

I get headaches after playing basketball. Is there a connection?

C.B., Aurora, Colorado

Are they worse when you lose? Seriously, what you describe are exercise-induced headaches. Some doctors think they're caused by a sudden increase in blood pressure, resulting in swollen blood vessels. Pretreat yourself with a pain reliever like Tylenol or Motrin half an hour before tip-off. Warm up so your body can adjust to the faster blood circulation, and try to take breaks. If the pain continues, see a doctor. Don't panic, but persistent headaches could mean a tumor or internal bleeding.

Final Exam

However, don't bank on it. The fact that hardly anyone dies during strength training doesn't prove it can't happen. Franklin points out that the men at greatest risk of sudden death during exercise are middle-aged; most lifters are young. More of us older guys are lifting today, but when the studies I've cited in this story were put together, in the '80s and early '90s, you didn't find many gray-hairs in the weight room. If a middle-aged guy was exercising, he was most likely running, riding a bike, or swatting at a fuzzy yellow ball.

But now we do have a substantial population of middle-aged men in health clubs, and we know a few of them will do their final cooldowns at the county morgue. Franklin recently looked at exercise-related deaths at a major chain of health clubs. Using swipe-card data, he tallied 183 million gym visits in the study period, during which time 71 members died while working out. It's not known what the deceased were doing at the fatal moment, so we can't draw many definitive conclusions.

But Franklin did find two interesting trends in the data: The average age of club members was 32. The average age of the 71 who died was 53. The 71 also averaged just two trips to the club per month. It's possible they were exercising outside the gym, but Franklin doubts it. If they had been, most of them would probably still be alive.

And that's the most reasonable conclusion one can draw about death by exercise: The best way to avoid it is to exercise. "The person who's at greatest risk of an exercise death is the person with known or hidden coronary artery disease who is habitually sedentary—a couch potato, all year round," says Franklin.

You don't need to turn into a marathoner. (Look what happened to Pheidippides.) But you should work out frequently; many studies have shown that the overall amount of time you spend up and moving matters.

Some endurance exercise is fine, if you like it. Strength training is probably more than fine—it specifically prepares your body for the shock of sudden, strenuous exertion, such as shoveling snow, which is most likely to kill you if your body isn't ready for it.

We can't attach any sort of dose-response number to weight lifting as a preventive to sudden death, but we do know it's pretty hard to kill yourself while doing it. For ex-

ample, if you assumed that every death recorded at the health clubs occurred during strength training, you'd still end up with just one fatality for every 2.5 million exercise sessions, which is lower than the one in 1.5 million that shows up in older studies of mostly aerobic exercisers.

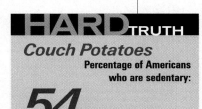

HARDTRUTH

Couch Potatoes

Percentage of Americans who are sedentary:

54

But any time you exercise strenuously, on the road or in the squat rack, you're taking on a small risk of a big problem. "It's like investing in the stock market," says Thompson. "You're putting your money down, looking for a long-term gain. But you could put your money in WorldCom and lose it all. There's a risk to everything."

BY IAN SMITH, M.D.

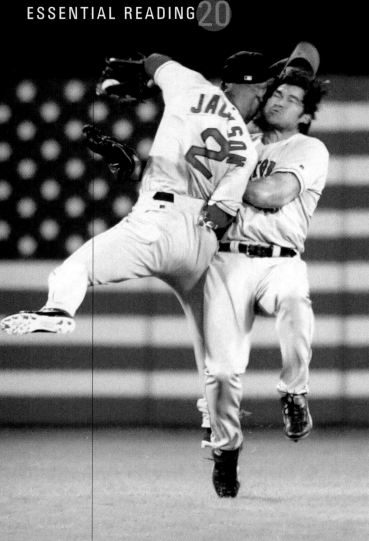

Your buddy hits the deck screaming. Do you know what to do? Our *Men's Health* team doctor tells you how to take charge when the blood flows

Any baller has been there. Somebody goes down, play stops, heads turn. If he stays down, there's that moment: Should we do something? (Then there are two other moments: Saying, "Walk it off," and if he can't, asking someone on the sidelines, "You in? We need one.")

Blood makes it more interesting. A lump is fascinating. A crooked limb, gross and fascinating. If you're a doctor, then it's time to go to work. That's where I come in.

I've seen my share of injuries, on the field and in the ER. I've even suffered a few myself. I know what to do. This chapter is your crash course in sideline first aid—the basics on blood, bruises, and breaks. So next time somebody goes down, you can step up while others stand back. You in?

A Healthy Dose of Sports Medicine

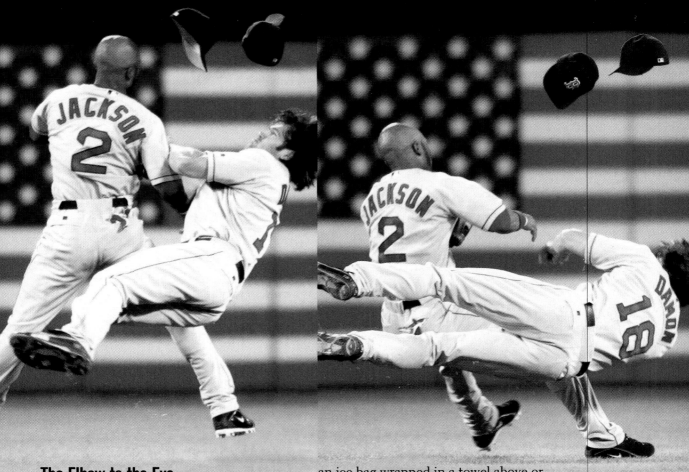

The Elbow to the Eye

LIKELY SPORTS: BASKETBALL, FOOTBALL, BAR FIGHT

First, be calm. Tell him to get his hands away from his eye—hold him down if you have to. Stop any bleeding around the eye with firm, gentle pressure, ideally using gauze or cotton balls—but a cleanish sweatshirt is fine. (See "Red Alert" on page 182.) When the bleeding is under control, apply an ice bag wrapped in a towel above or below the eye.

THE EXAM

Look for anything askew—specifically if the eye is sitting at a strange angle. Puffiness is expected, but bleeding, twitching, or a pronounced lump on the bony ridge around the eye is really bad. Compare the injured side of the face with the other side.

Trace gently, with your thumb and index finger, the bone structure around the eye. Check for spots where the bones can be moved.

Ask simple questions. Are things blurry? Any flashes of light? Does it feel as if something is in his eye?

Tell him to follow your finger as you slowly draw the letter H in the air 6 inches in front of him.

GO TO THE ER?

Yes, if his eyes don't follow your finger, there's bleeding within the eye, or he answers "yes" to any of the above questions. His vision is at stake. The eyes are surrounded by crucial muscles, nerves, and bones. Never take chances.

No, if his eyesight is okay, there are no pronounced lumps, and nothing looks cockeyed.

My Advice: Don't hold ice directly on the eye, but on the bone above or below, and for no more than 10 minutes at a time. Any longer might injure sensitive tissues. I saw one guy who took an elbow in the eye going for a rebound. He was seeing double and couldn't complete the H test. We sent him and his hot-pink eye to the ER, where they diagnosed him with a ruptured eye muscle. (It looks as bad as it sounds.) Without surgery, his vision might never have recovered.

The Audible Knee Pop

LIKELY SPORTS: SKIING, FOOTBALL, BASKETBALL, SOFTBALL, SOCCER, TENNIS

First, find a warm place for him to sit and elevate his knee—even if he doesn't feel any pain, which is possible. Arrange for rest, ice, compression, and elevation (RICE), the standard treatment for many joint and muscle injuries. (See "Rice Check" on opposite page.) This is critical in the early treatment, because the knee will swell anywhere from 2 to 12 hours after the injury. Give him some Motrin or Tylenol.

THE EXAM

Hold his foot in one hand, and support the calf with the other. Gently and very slowly

Red Alert

Stop the bleeding

Direct, even pressure on bleeding works—but most people don't keep the pressure on long enough. For at least 10 minutes, resist the temptation to peek. Elevate the wound above the level of the heart to reduce bloodflow. Use a compress directly on the wound. (A clean, heavy gauze pad is best, but a T-shirt or sock—the cleaner the better—works fine.) Sometimes this doesn't work. You can further reduce bloodflow by pressing on a major artery heading toward the injured spot. Feel for the arterial pulse, and push down on it, against the bone, while maintaining pressure on the wound for 2 minutes. If this doesn't stop the bleeding, head to a hospital.

The four pressure points: the middle inside of the upper arm (the brachial artery); the wrist just before the base of the thumb (radial artery); the groin (femoral artery); and the back of the knee (popliteal artery).

move the knee to see if it has a normal range of motion compared with the uninjured leg—bend it, then extend it, then move the lower leg from side to side. If you're careful, this is a safe way to assess damage, but leave it to a real doctor if you're unsure. A sharp pain indicates damage to a ligament or cartilage.

Ask what he was doing when it popped. If it happened during a pivot movement or a quick stop or sudden turn, it may be a torn ACL, the anterior cruciate ligament. About 100,000 people tear their ACLs each year. If the knee starts "locking" or "catching" and is difficult to walk on, it may be damage to the cartilage in the knee joint.

GO TO THE ER?

Yes, if he can't stand because of the pain, or if there's swelling, loss of mobility, or limping.

No, if he can get around and endure the discomfort. He should go home and use the RICE treatment to keep the swelling down. And he should schedule a doctor appointment to assess the damage.

My Advice: After any kind of knee injury, see a doctor before resuming sports. Activity on an injured ACL can damage the cartilage in the knee, creating more problems.

The Line Drive to the Head

LIKELY SPORT: SOFTBALL

First, scalp wounds bleed profusely. If it's just a cut, apply gentle pressure until the bleeding is under control. If the wound seems deep or if there's excessive blood,

Rice Check

Reduce the swelling

For pulled muscles and joint injuries, the RICE treatment is standard—and essential—for a speedy recovery.

Rest is critical. Aggravating the injured area leads to more pain and inflammation.

Ice should be applied immediately. It relieves pain and reduces swelling by slowing bloodflow to the injury. Apply it for 15 minutes on, 15 minutes off. After 72 hours, stop ice treatment so blood can heal the injury.

Compression bandages (like Ace) also reduce swelling. Don't wrap too tightly. What's too tight? If you start feeling a numbness or heaviness in your extremities or, even worse, if the skin color starts to change to a bluish gray.

Elevation also reduces swelling. Keep the injured body part above the level of your heart. Sitting on the couch with your leg propped up isn't enough—you've got to lie down. (Tell your wife it's doctor's orders.)

don't touch it; drive your friend to the ER. Take any head injury seriously—a concussion or cracked skull bones are possible.

THE EXAM

Ask him his name, the day, and a detail about the game.

Look in his eyes to see if he's focused. That's it. That was just for show, because you don't mess around with head injuries. Bleeding, headache, dizziness, vision or hearing problems, vomiting—note all symptoms so you can tell them to the doctor.

(continued on page 186)

Gory Days

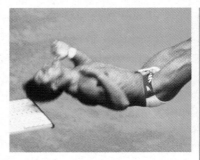

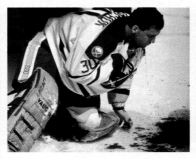

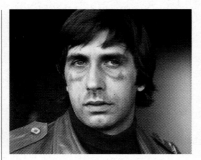

We rank the greatest hits and hurts of all time

10. Banging the Head Board

Greg Louganis was off balance in his take-off at the 1988 Olympics, causing his head to collide with the diving board. With four temporary sutures, Louganis returned and went on to win two gold medals.

Time on the DL: 30 minutes

9. Y.A.'s Moment of Clarity

New York Giants quarterback Y.A. Tittle took a sack from the Pittsburgh Steelers' John Baker in 1964 that merely bruised his ribs. But Tittle estimates he was knocked cold at least five times in his 16-year career.

Time on the DL: 1 week

8. Don't Eat the Cherry Sno-Cone

A pileup in front of the goal ended with Buffalo Sabres goalie Clint Malarchuk severing his jugular vein on a skate. Malarchuk skated away but needed 60 stitches to close the 6-inch slice.

Time on the DL: 11 days

7. The Original Mad Cow Disease

A novice bullfighter in Guaderrama, Spain, made a crucial misstep, and a bull gored him with its horns. Though this happened in 1972, we suspect the bullfighter still has trouble putting it behind him.

Time on the DL: Some wounds will never heal.

6. "Eeww, what's that taste?"

Witness the aftermath of L.A. Laker Kermit Washington's right hand colliding with Houston Rocket Rudy Tomjanovich's face. The blow broke bones in Rudy T.'s face, dislodged his skull, and caused spinal fluid to leak into his mouth. Five surgeries later, he was cleared to play.

Time on the DL: 5 months

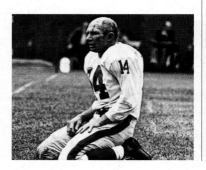

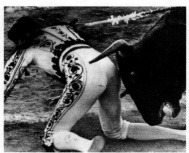

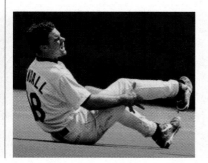

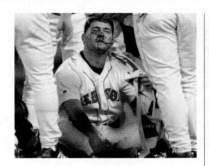

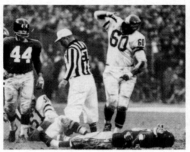

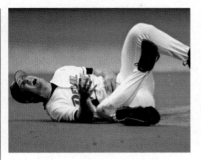

5. Taking It on the Shin

Pittsburgh Pirates catcher Jason Kendall snagged the side of the bag trying to beat out a bunt in a game in 1999. He dislocated his right ankle, and his tibia (shinbone) pierced the skin, so the wound filled with dirt. After surgery and a titanium implant to repair two torn ligaments, he returned to the field.

Time on the DL: 8 months

4. The Boston Beaned Play

In 2000, Yankee Ryan Thompson hit a line drive that bounded off Boston Red Sox pitcher Bryce Florie's face. The ball fractured his cheekbone, his nose, and his eye socket in three places, and damaged his retina.

Time on the DL: 10 months

3. Insult Plus Injury Equals History

While trying to catch a pass, Frank Gifford of the New York Giants was blindsided by Philadelphia linebacker Chuck Bednarik. The Eagles won and Bednarik celebrated as Gifford lay out cold with a severe concussion that kept him unconscious for 36 hours.

Time on the DL: 1 year

2. The Least Funny Humerus Incident

Tampa Bay Devil Rays pitcher Tony Saunders broke his left arm in midpitch to Texas Ranger Juan Gonzalez in 1999. Saunders suffered a career-ending spiral break of the humerus (the bone in the upper arm), his second in 15 months. Doctors suspect that the torque and force of pitching may have been the cause.

Time on the DL: Eternity

1. The Break Heard Round the World

Quarterback Joe Theisman earned the number-one spot in the Hall of Pain with a compound fracture of his right leg during a Monday night game in 1985. Theisman's career ended after New York Giants linebackers Lawrence Taylor and Gary Reasons piled on top of him.

Time on the DL: Eternity

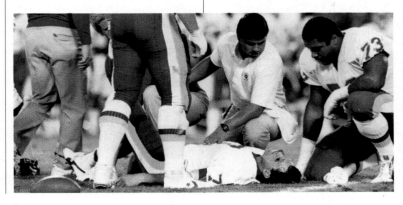

GO TO THE ER?

Yes. No exceptions. A blow to the head can cause internal bleeding that won't produce any visible, immediate symptoms. But hours, even a day later, he could have a seizure, go into a coma, and die. Anytime a blow causes external bleeding, instant headache, vision changes, or loss of consciousness, he may need a CT scan to look for bleeding in his brain.

My Advice: Most people who suffer concussions never lose consciousness. That doesn't mean there's no injury. A recent study in the *Journal of the American Medical Association* shows that you're far more susceptible to another concussion for 7 to 10 days after the first one. When I was in college, I knew a varsity hockey player who was seemingly destined for the NHL. A couple of years after graduation, he told me doctors had forbidden him to play. He'd suffered concussions throughout his career but continued to go back on the ice to take a pounding. Soon he was having memory problems. Any more hockey, docs said, would put him at risk of permanent brain injury.

The Injury Report

Turf toe and other sports-page terms deciphered

Cauliflower Ear A deformed ear caused by repeated blows, usually suffered by boxers or wrestlers. A blood clot develops under the skin, or the skin is stripped away from the structural cartilage, causing it to die and resemble your least favorite vegetable.

Groin Pull The adductor muscles—in the inner thigh— are overextended and torn. A thorough warmup and stretch will help prevent it. Keep the adductors strong by doing squats and lunges.

High Ankle Sprain A regular sprain happens when your foot is flat and rolls to the outside. With the high kind of sprain, you land on your toes and then roll. This separates your tibia and fibula and sprains the ligaments in between. Non-football players are more likely to get one running down the stairs or stepping off the curb. Recovery is longer than with a regular sprain.

Hip Pointer When that bony point on your hip gets smashed by a helmet, the muscle and bone become bruised. That's one kind of hip pointer. Jumping and kicking can also cause the muscle to pull away from the bone, causing another type. Spend 5 minutes warming up, unless you want 2 to 10 weeks of inactivity.

Stinger One shoulder goes down and your head gets forced the other way, stretching the brachial plexus nerves in your neck. You're in pain, and your arm goes dead for a few minutes. It's a common injury in professional sports, caused by poor tackling or being upended and coming down on the side of your head. Weekend quarterbacks shouldn't expect to get this one.

Turf Toe The big-toe joint gets jammed and sprained, and it's hard to walk on. The injury is common among pro football players, and unforgiving artificial turf is the main cause.

The Scattered Chiclets

LIKELY SPORTS: HOCKEY, FOOTBALL

First, grab some ice, and apply it to the mouth and gums. Keep his head tilted forward, so blood and teeth won't go down his throat. Have the other guys collect any broken teeth. Wash them in cold milk or water, or grab someone's contact lens saline solution and cover the teeth in it. Handle them as little as possible, and do not touch the roots. If he can, have your buddy put the teeth back in their sockets; if not, leave them in the wash solution.

GO TO THE ER?

Yes, right now, because teeth can be saved, especially if you act quickly. He'll also need an x-ray to see if the jaw is fractured, and may require stitches to stop the bleeding in his mouth.

My Advice: Tell him not to freak out. Oral surgeons and plastic surgeons can work miracles these days. And before he goes back out there, make sure he splurges for a face mask.

The Turned Ankle

LIKELY SPORT: YOU NAME IT

First, keep him on the ground. Resist the urge to take the shoe off to see how bad it is—leaving it laced can keep swelling down until you have some ice ready.

THE EXAM

Support his foot with a ball, a cooler, anything that keeps it higher than his head.

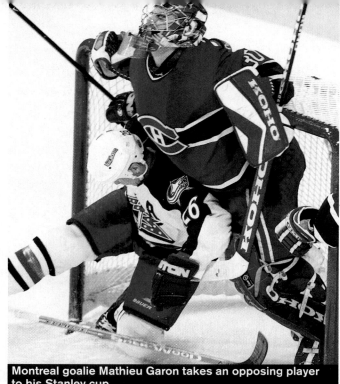

Montreal goalie Mathieu Garon takes an opposing player to his Stanley cup.

Tell him to rotate his foot in the normal range of motion.

Look for any limitations or excruciating pain in the various positions. If he can't move the ankle at all, bones could be broken.

GO TO THE ER?

Yes, if there's extreme tenderness directly on the ankle (bruising may not occur right away, but if there is any, it's a sign he needs a doctor's care), or if he can't put weight on it. He should get an x-ray. A sprain means the ligaments holding the joint together are stretched or torn. But in many cases, there are fractures as well.

No, if he's able to put weight on it without sharp pain, and the discomfort dissipates. He should still use RICE treatment at home.

My Advice: Keep your sneakers fresh. No, not the smell. New ones every few months will help cushion the extreme pressure put on your ankles every time you step or jump. There are no solid statistics showing that high-tops prevent sprains, but I think they help. The American Academy of Orthopedic Surgeons says that every day, 25,000 people sprain an ankle.

The Shot to the Balls

LIKELY SPORTS: SOFTBALL, SOCCER

First, give the poor guy a minute or 8. Then tell him to inspect the damage. The testicles are surrounded by lymphatic and blood vessels, and swelling can occur disturbingly fast.

Stay Off the DL

Fix your weakness before you break it

Chest and Shoulders

The test: Hold your arms out in front of your chest with palms facing down. Keeping your elbows at shoulder height, pull your arms back until your hands are right in front of your chest.

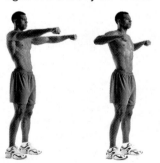

You should be able to perform the motion without any pain. Otherwise, there may be damage to muscles around the shoulder, making you prone to upper-body injuries like rotator-cuff tears.

If you fail: Place your hand against a wall with your arm at shoulder height. Lean forward and bend your elbow, stretching the pectoral and shoulder muscles. "This stretch puts your muscles through all the ranges of motion and also gets the nervous system coordinated so it knows what to do when you start to load weight," says Ken Kinakin, D.C., author of *Optimal Muscle Training*.

Hips and Back

The test: In a seated position, grab your leg below the

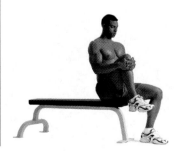

knee and raise it toward your chest. If you can't lift your knee above a 45-degree angle, you're asking for a groin pull or back strain.

If you fail: Lie on your back. Place the bottom of one foot flat against a wall, knee bent 90 degrees. Push on the wall with the bottom of your foot for 8 seconds, then place your hand on your thigh above your kneecap and push against your knee for 8 seconds. "A lot of times, there's strength imbalance between the front and the back," says Kinakin.

Hamstrings

The test: Lie in a doorway with one leg up on the doorframe and the other one flat on the floor. If you can't straighten both legs, the next snap you hear might not come from your Rice Krispies.

THE EXAM (He can do this himself, okay?)

Look for swelling or bruising.

Feel for tender spots.

Apply ice (wrapped in a towel) for 10 minutes, then take it off for 20 minutes. The skin in that area is thin, so don't put ice directly on it.

Drink some water or a sports drink, and urinate to make sure the stream is normal in strength, color, and direction.

GO TO THE ER?

Yes, if he notices bruising or a dark (blood-tinged) or weak urine stream, or if swelling doesn't subside in 24 hours.

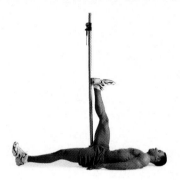

If you fail: "Any aerobic exercise is good to warm up the lower extremities," says Ken Schaecher, manager of physical therapy at the Oklahoma Center for Athletes. Spending 10 minutes on a stair machine before your regular workout will help prevent damage.

Ankles

The test: Stand on a step with your heels hanging off the edge. Lower your heels 45 degrees, then raise them 90 degrees so that you're up on your toes. If you can't raise and lower them to a 45-degree angle, you're a prime candidate for a sprain.

If you fail: Strengthen your calf muscles by practicing the above test. Once you can complete 10 repetitions, repeat the move holding dumbbells. Adding resistance to standing calf raises can prevent ankle injuries, as can stretching the muscle.

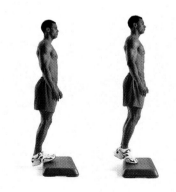

Knees

The test: Ask a trainer at your gym to help you determine your one-rep maximum for leg extensions and leg curls. If your leg-curl max, which measures hamstring strength, isn't 65 percent of your leg-extension max, which measures quadriceps strength, you could be prone to injury. Orthopedic surgeons live off these imbalances.

If you fail: Do more leg curls than squats. "In most individuals who are not elite athletes, their hamstrings are significantly weaker than their quadriceps—much less than two-thirds," says Scott Lephart, Ph.D., director of research at the University of Pittsburgh Medical Center's center for sports medicine. "If you exercise your hamstrings more than your quadriceps, you'll help even out that imbalance."

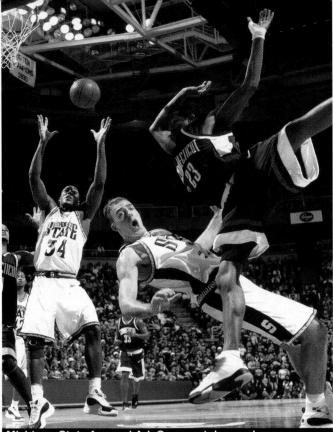

Michigan State forward A.J. Granger takes a charge, pays with pain.

eral socks tied together. (Tie him after the exam.)

THE EXAM

Touch his hand and arm to make sure the skin isn't turning cold, indicating a circulation problem. Gently, now.

Poke or touch him in various spots from the shoulder down his arm to the fingers to see if he feels it; a lack of sensation may indicate nerve damage.

Ask him to wiggle his fingers.

Give him something lightweight (like a water bottle), and see if he's able to lift it.

GO TO THE ER?

Yes, but there's no need to break the speed limit. This type of injury isn't life threatening, but it can hurt like hell. A doctor needs to evaluate damage to the collarbone and stabilizing ligaments.

My Advice: I've just described a separated shoulder, not a dislocated shoulder. What's the difference? A separation means the ligaments that hold the clavicle to the shoulder blade are completely or partially torn. In a dislocation, the upper-arm bone (the humerus) comes out of the shoulder socket. If he can't move his arm or the pain is excruciating, it's probably dislocated. With a separation, he'll be able to move it, but it'll still hurt.

The Snapped Collarbone

LIKELY SPORTS: CYCLING, FOOTBALL

First, just get him off the field. (Or scrape him off the road.) He shouldn't try to move the arm, but then, he won't want to. Immobi-

No, if everything's working and he's feeling better.

My Advice: Feeling light-headed or nauseated is common, so don't be alarmed if he vomits. The exact cause of the nausea is unclear, but it probably has to do with our nervous system and involuntary reflexes. It's true—everything does lead to our balls.

The Separated Shoulder

LIKELY SPORTS: FOOTBALL, SKIING, CYCLING, ROCK CLIMBING

First, keep the elbow bent 90 degrees and the arm flush against his abdomen. Wrap his arm against his body, using a shirt or sev-

lize it with a makeshift sling. If the bones move around, they can puncture or compress a lung or artery. You don't want to see this.

THE EXAM

Trace your finger gently over the collarbone to feel the fracture. But he won't let you, so . . .

GO TO THE ER?

Uh, yeah. Some broken clavicles come through the skin, increasing the chance of an infection. In that case, hurry. But in a typical case, there's nothing a doctor can do but fit him with a sling to immobilize the upper body so the bone can heal.

My Advice: Orthopedic surgeons joke that with collarbone fractures they just "slap on a Band-Aid and send them home," because often there's little to do but order a splint and a sling. Of course, it's not that simple. Most collarbone breaks are in the middle of the bone. But a "distal third" fracture, close to the shoulder, must be monitored by a physician. I once had a guy come into my office with a complaint about another part of his body, but when I examined him, I noticed his clavicle had a knob the size of a golf ball. It had been broken in college, and he'd been put in a splint, but when the pain faded, he tossed the splint. The grotesque bone nodule was his lifelong reward for playing doctor.

The Twanged Hamstring

LIKELY SPORTS: SOFTBALL, SOCCER, FOOTBALL, BASKETBALL

First, send him to the sidelines, and get some ice. He can't walk off a pulled hamstring; he'll just reinjure it. He needs RICE treatment as quickly as possible—minutes matter. Wrap the thigh with a compressive dressing like an Ace bandage, which will help keep the swelling down.

THE EXAM

Listen for screams. Pain is the first indicator.

Run your hand down the back of the thigh, and make sure it feels like a long, smooth muscle. A tight ball is a sign of a bad pull or possible tear or rupture.

GO TO THE ER?

No, usually. Most of the time this treatment can be handled on the sideline, in the trainer's room, or at home. Mild to moderate pulls are painful, but the person can still stand and walk.

Drink Up

As the NFL preseason shows us every year, thirsty guys rapidly turn into dead guys. Dehydration can also cause dizziness, nausea, vomiting, high body temperatures, rapid heartbeat, and a tendency to mix stripes and plaids. To avoid all that, add the temperature to the relative humidity. If the sum is greater than 159, drink up. David Janda, director of the Institute for Preventative Sports Medicine, advises you guzzle . . .

2 cups of water—2 hours before your workout

6 ounces—every 45 minutes of your workout

3 cups—for every pound you lost during the workout

Yes, if the pain is excruciating and the person can't stand or walk. If the muscle or muscles are ruptured or extensively torn, they may require surgical repair.

My Advice: In a day or so, he may see a bruise form on the back of the thigh or near the knee as the blood from the injury drains down the leg. The key to recovery is rest. If he comes back too soon, he'll reinjure it. A mild pull can take just 7 to 10 days to heal, but severe cases can take weeks or months.

The Jammed Finger

LIKELY SPORTS: BASKETBALL, FOOTBALL, VOLLEYBALL

First, don't tell him to tape the bad finger to its neighbor. That's for pros playing for millions. He just might aggravate the injury. And don't yank on his finger, thinking you'll pop it back into place. There's too great a chance you'll damage soft tissues, which could easily result in permanent impairment and deformity—and really, isn't your buddy deformed enough?

THE EXAM

Compare it with the same finger on the other hand. Is it crooked or pointing the wrong way?

Apply ice, and have him elevate the hand with the injured finger to reduce inflammation.

Wait a few minutes, then have him try to move the finger slightly. If he can without severe pain, send him back into the game. If the finger doesn't move easily or the pain gets worse, it's time to go on the DL.

GO TO THE ER?

Nah. But if swelling, stiffness, and pain last longer than 48 hours, have the finger x-rayed to see if it's broken.

My Advice: A typical jammed finger isn't a broken finger. It's an injury to the ligaments and/or tendons surrounding the middle knuckle in the finger—that is, the proximal interphalangeal, or PIP, joint, if you want to dazzle the bystanders.

Road Rash

LIKELY SPORT: CYCLING

First, clean the wound with water from a squirt bottle—the pressure helps wash away dirt and dead skin. If he's gushing blood, use the nearest and cleanest cloth to stop it;

This pileup had five Down Under footballers feeling scummy all over.

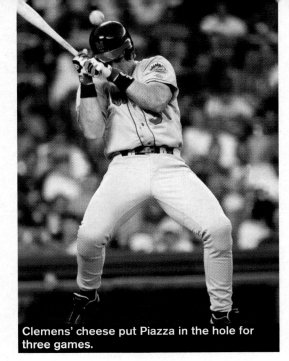

Clemens' cheese put Piazza in the hole for three games.

breathable natural fibers are the best choice.

THE EXAM

Look at it and say, "Ooh, that's gotta smart."

Wash it (let him do it, if he can reach) at home with a mild soap like Ivory.

Cover it with an antibiotic cream and breathable sterile dressing. Change the dressing every couple of days, and keep the wound moist until it has healed.

GO TO THE ER?

Yes, even though he may think that's an overreaction. Some stitches might make healing smoother, and the doctor may recommend a tetanus shot if your buddy hasn't had a booster within the past 10 years.

My Advice: Antibiotic ointments like Mederma or Neosporin seem to make wounds heal more smoothly, though I haven't seen conclusive evidence. Make sure to apply it as soon as possible after the injury.

The Smashed Nose

LIKELY SPORTS: FOOTBALL, BASKETBALL, HOCKEY, BAR FIGHT

First, hold a gauze pad or towel firmly to his nose, and have him lean forward slightly to prevent him from swallowing blood. Keep the pad there longer than you'd think—check underneath in 10 or 15 minutes to see if it's stopped.

THE EXAM

Check the bloodflow every 15 minutes; if he's still gushing after 45 minutes, it's probably broken.

Look at the nose and see if it's crooked, or if bruises are forming under his eyes.

Ask if he's having trouble breathing—beyond the stuffiness of a nose full of drying blood.

GO TO THE ER?

Yes, if it looks like a break. Unless he's looking for added character (it works for Owen Wilson), it's best to let a doc set it. One clue it's broken: a grape-size swelling inside the nostril, alongside the nasal bone.

My Advice: One of the best ways to stop a bleeding nose is to soak strips of gauze in saline (salty) solution or in an antibiotic ointment, then pack them gently into the nostrils for up to 30 minutes. If that doesn't work, go to a hospital.

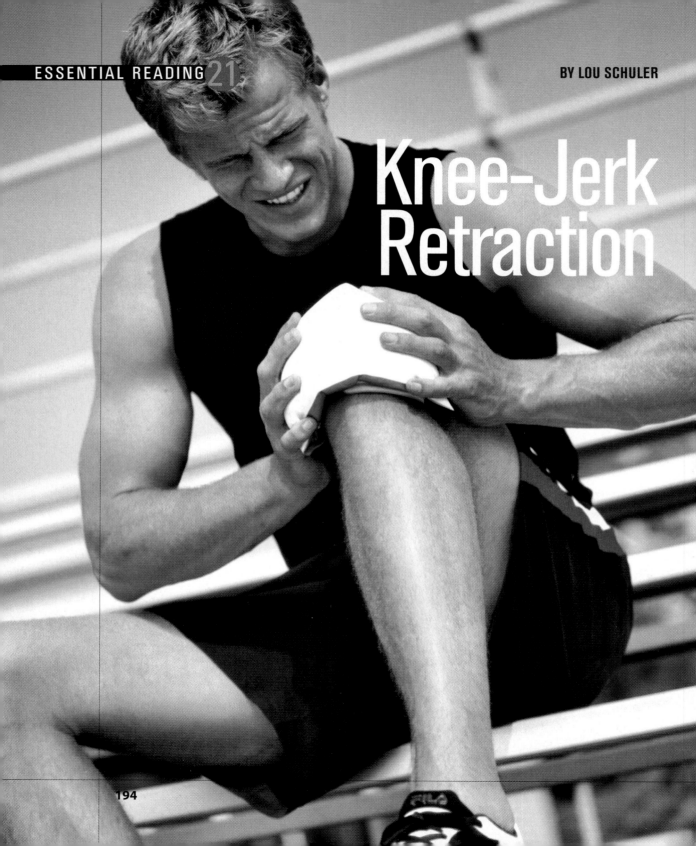

BY LOU SCHULER

Knee-Jerk Retraction

Show your joints who's chief, and banish the pain for good

What made me stronger damn near crippled me. It happened like this: I'd flown to Boston to work on a basketball story. Up to that point, I'd played pickup ball once or twice a week for 10 years with knee pain that I managed with elastic braces, ice, and occasional doses of ibuprofen. I played twice in one day in Boston, then returned on a cramped plane the next morning.

My knees were never the same. I found myself walking downcourt, conserving my jumps—anything to avoid jarring my pain-wracked knees. Even after I quit playing ball, the pain was constant. If I got down on the floor to pick up after my kids, I couldn't get back up without using both hands, grunting like a sumo wrestler on his wedding night. I couldn't sit for any length of time without my knees aching.

That last fact forced me to deal with the problem. I had committed to driving my wife and kids to a family reunion, a round-trip of close to 2,000 miles and about 32 hours. Since I couldn't sit with bent knees longer than half an hour, the thought of 64 half hours behind the wheel seemed like a death march.

All of which I related to Brian Halpern, M.D., just 5 days before the trip. Halpern is a physician at the Hospital for Special Surgery in Manhattan and author of *The Knee Crisis Handbook* (Rodale Inc., 2003). He figured out the problem in less time than

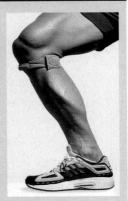

PAINkiller

Weak-Kneed

My knees kill me after hoops. Do those stretchy bands some guys wear below the knee actually work?
P.Y., Denver

It's technically called an infrapatellar strap, but you can call it a knee strap. They were made fashionable by Michael Jordan, among others. The bands are intended to reduce or eliminate pain by stabilizing tendons and more evenly distributing the pressure across the knee. There's not much scientific evidence indicating that they work, but there's plenty of anecdotal testimony. It's your call on how you want to spend your $15. If you do, though, at least look cool. Get a black one.

it took me to explain why I was there: inflexible and unbalanced quadriceps muscles. I wondered why I hadn't deduced this on my own, being the Muscle Guy and all. But Halpern assured me that few of the weak-kneed—fitness professional and civilian alike—can decode their own aches.

So that was lesson number one: Don't diagnose yourself. Here are three more.

If It Feels Bad, Don't Do It

I know why it took me so long to address my knee problems. I didn't want a doctor to tell me the obvious: Stop playing basketball. If your knees hurt, the worst thing you can do is continue a pain-causing activity.

None of this means you have to stop moving. The key is to unload the knee joint, but remain active, since inactivity can lead to weight gain and more stress on your knees.

Inaction plan: Work your knee through any painless range of motion that's possible, even if it's only a few degrees. Your body will do whatever it can to "splint" an injury, tensing muscles surrounding a joint to keep it immobilized. So if you simply lie on your back and bend and straighten your aching knees without causing further pain, you'll relieve the tension in the muscles. (Cycling is even better, provided it doesn't hurt.) Gentle movement also speeds up the body's healing processes, encouraging nutrient-rich blood and the joints' natural lubricants to flow into the area.

Work All Your Muscles

In *The Knee Crisis Handbook,* Halpern tells of a competitive cyclist suffering severe knee pain. His outer-thigh muscles were much stronger than those of the inner thigh.

Most sports and exercise routines favor some muscles over others, and the imbalance can force the kneecap out of alignment, literally rubbing it the wrong way. Runners often have strong, tight hamstrings and calves but weak quadriceps. Then there's the lifter with bulging quadriceps but relatively weak hamstrings.

The Knee-Injury Decoder

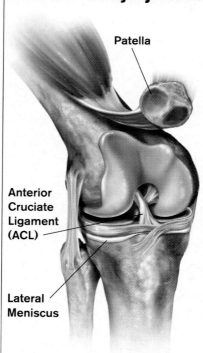

Patella

Anterior
Cruciate
Ligament
(ACL)

Lateral
Meniscus

Knee pain comes in many varieties. There's the writhing-on-the-ground kind, the annoying-limp kind, and the kind that makes you rub your knee all day long while muttering darkly. Don't despair—all of them can be fixed, with enough time and the right diagnosis. Start here.

THE PAIN: You hear a pop, or sense that something has snapped. Your knee swells within 2 hours, there is intense pain, and your leg buckles if you try to put weight on it.

Most likely: A stretched or torn anterior cruciate ligament (ACL), one of two ligaments that form an X within the joint.

The fix: A complete tear usually means surgery and 4 to 6 months of rehabilitation. For a sprain (it's stretched but not torn), figure 4 to 12 weeks of rehab, depending on the severity of the injury.

THE PAIN: Your knee clicks, sometimes locks, hurts on stairs, and really hurts when you get up from a low chair.

Most likely: A torn or worn-down meniscus, a cartilage pad in the knee joint. A worn-down meniscus can lose shock absorption. When it's damaged, pieces can get caught between bones, causing the clicking

The classic recommended acceptable strength ratio is 3:2, which means your quadriceps should be no more than 50 percent stronger than your hamstrings.

Self-test 1: Figure out your ratio by doing a maximum-weight leg curl and leg extension with each leg. Then simply divide your quadriceps strength by your hamstring strength. Do this for both legs, if there's a strength difference. The

big problems start when your hamstrings are only half as strong as your quadriceps—a 2:1 strength ratio.

Self-test 2: Gauge imbalances between inner and outer thighs by watching yourself in a mirror while doing squats. If your knees buckle inward when you use heavier weights, your inner thighs are stronger. If your knees drift outward, you're outer-thigh dominant.

sound or causing the bones to lock in place.

The fix: Small tears can sometimes repair themselves with 4 to 6 weeks of physical therapy. Larger tears can be repaired surgically, meaning 4 weeks on crutches and perhaps several weeks of rehab.

THE PAIN: The front of your knee hurts, and it's especially tender just below the kneecap. Climbing stairs and getting up from a chair both hurt.

Most likely: Patellar tendinitis, also called "jumper's knee," caused by overuse. It's inflammation of the tendon (technically a ligament) that connects the kneecap to the shinbone. If you play through knee pain, it'll never heal.

The fix: Rest, stretching, and strength exercises—beef up your thigh muscles with leg extensions or leg presses. To reduce the strain on the patellar tendon, wear shoe inserts from a drugstore and an infrapatellar strap (worn below the kneecap) or Neoprene sleeve.

THE PAIN: It's all on the front of the knee, under or around the kneecap. It's worse when lunging or squatting, or after sitting for a long time.

Most likely: Patellofemoral syndrome, also called "runner's knee." Tight tendons (such as the iliotibial band, on the side of the leg) or muscles (especially the hamstrings) cause the kneecap to slip off track and grind against the thighbone. Untreated, this can damage the cartilage protecting the joint, and may lead to osteoarthritis.

The fix: Lots of strength exercises (usually the innermost part of the quadriceps is weaker than the outer parts), stretching (especially the hamstrings), and regular doses of glucosamine and chondroitin sulfate supplements for cartilage repair.

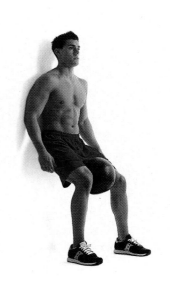
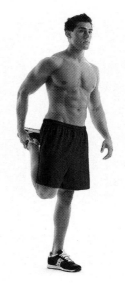
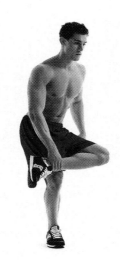

Strong medicine: This move will help you build balanced strength. Put a basketball or medicine ball between your knees, and stand with your back flat against a wall. Your feet should be parallel and about 24 inches from the wall. Squeeze the ball with your knees, then slide down the wall until your thighs are about 45 degrees from vertical. Hold for 15 seconds, then push back up the wall. Repeat nine times, rest 60 seconds, and do another set of 10 repetitions.

WALL SLIDE

If that's easy (and painless), move your feet out and slide down the wall until your thighs are parallel to the floor. Don't let your knees go past your toes. Increase the length of time you hold the stretch to 60 seconds. Repeat five times, and do two or three sets.

Stretch All Day Long

After I saw Halpern, I started stretching my quadriceps almost every waking hour. On my vacation, I got out of the car at every restroom break and stretched. I got through the trip with virtually no knee pain. After workouts, stretching eased my stiffness.

My knees aren't exactly cured—I still

Wrap It Up

Tape fixes everything. A study published in the *British Medical Journal* found that therapeutic knee tape, when worn for 3 weeks, reduces knee pain caused by osteoarthritis by as much as 63 percent for most people. Study author Rana Hinman, Ph.D., surmises that the tape "changes the position of the kneecap and thus relieves pressure behind it." The tape, which has soft and rigid layers, is available at pharmacies, but see a physiotherapist to have your knee assessed. Those without osteoarthritis can also reduce pain by wearing tape during activity. Just remove it afterward.

can't do full squats or lunges—but for big chunks of the day, they feel normal.

Flex plan: The standing quad stretch is easy and made a near-instant impact on my knee health. Pull the heel of one foot up to your butt, keeping your thighs parallel. Rest your opposite hand against a wall, or keep that hand at your side to develop better strength and balance in your feet and ankles.

FIGURE-4 STRETCH

Another favorite is the standing figure-4 stretch. Grab something for balance, cross your left ankle over your right knee, and drop down until you feel a stretch in your left gluteals. Hold all stretches 15 to 30 seconds, and start with your tighter side.

PEAK
performance

Shower Power

A recent study from the University of Otago in New Zealand found that a postworkout sauna impaired the performance of competitive rowers 2 days later. On the other hand, another recent study showed that a cold plunge right after a workout can help you recover faster. But the best strategy might be a combination of hot and cold "contrast baths" after a workout, says Mark Verstegen, a trainer of elite athletes and author of *Core Performance* (Rodale Inc., 2004). You can do this in the shower, alternating between 3 minutes of hot and 1 minute of cold.

Save Your Knees

The first hint of aging often hits below the belt—in the knees. Keep your hinges strong with this exercise from Mike Caza, C.S.C.S. You'll need an exercise box or other low platform that can support your weight. Do 6 to 10 repetitions with each leg.

Power Lunge

With the box about 5 feet in front of you, stand with your feet hip-width apart and hold two light dumbbells at your sides. Step forward with your right leg, so that your right thigh ends up parallel to the floor and the knee is over your toes.

Now step onto the box with your left foot. Step down; repeat on the other side.

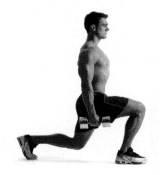

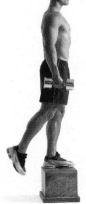

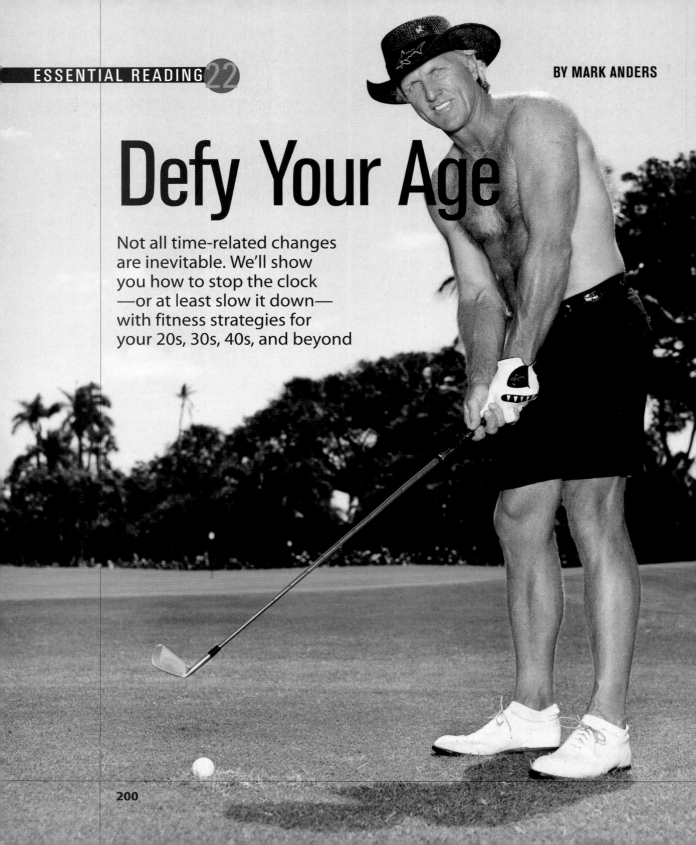

BY MARK ANDERS

Defy Your Age

Not all time-related changes
are inevitable. We'll show
you how to stop the clock
—or at least slow it down—
with fitness strategies for
your 20s, 30s, 40s, and beyond

Age 20 to 29: Grow, Show, and Go

Nature doesn't give a damn whether you live beyond the age of 25," says Leonard Hayflick, Ph.D., a professor emeritus at the University of California, San Francisco, and author of *How and Why We Age*. "Nature's only concern is that we live long enough to raise offspring to independence." That's why for most of human history, the average life expectancy has been about 20 years.

Of course, we've found ways to live longer, primarily by eradicating diseases. But the surest way to cheat death is to stack the game early. Think of your 20s as a decade of pregame practice. Invest a couple of hours of effort every week now, and it will save you a decades-long decline later.

The Changes
HORMONAL CHAOS

Your body is pumping out tons of human growth hormone (HGH) and testosterone, which leads to a peak in muscle mass sometime between ages 18 and 25, says Walter Thompson, Ph.D., a professor of kinesiology, health, and nutrition at Georgia State University in Atlanta. The bad part: It's only temporary.

The Fix

Feast on the flood. By the time you're 22 or 23, HGH production begins to decrease, dropping 2 to 5 percent each decade after that, silently stealing your strength. Build as much as you can now, and when you're 40 you can just maintain the brawn.

CREAKY KNEES

Researchers at Johns Hopkins University followed 1,321 former medical students and found that those who injured their knees as young adults were more than twice as likely to develop arthritis as they grew old.

The Fix

Stretch your hamstrings. Lack of flexibility in the hamstrings causes many knee problems. Avoid them with this hamstring stretch: Sit on the floor with your legs straight and spread a few feet apart. Bend your right leg and bring the foot to your left knee. Then try to touch both hands to your left foot. Hold the stretch for 20 to 30 seconds, then switch legs. Repeat three times every day.

Ease up on the cardio. Pounding the pavement too hard, too often can wear down the cartilage in your joints. So limit your running to no more than 4 days a week. Instead,

Time's Toll

The one-rep-maximum bench press for the average guy is . . .

6 percent more than his body weight in his 20s

7 percent less than his body weight in his 30s

16 percent less than his body weight in his 40s

25 percent less than his body weight in his 50s

32 percent less than his body weight in his 60s

The average man's absolute strength (the ratio of weight lifted to body weight) declines by 36 percent from his 20s to his 60s.

try a sport like basketball, in which you start and stop often. It's actually better for your cartilage than the repetitive pounding of jogging. Strength training can also strengthen cartilage, says Thompson.

THE FAT TIDE

During college, most guys eat like sumo wrestlers but burn off the extra calories playing sports, walking to class, chasing skirts, and just being generally active. After graduation, the feast continues—but without the physical activity. "From the day of graduation, most men start gaining weight," says Thompson. "Before long, you're sitting at your desk and you're 25 pounds overweight."

The Fix

Travel east for healthy eats. Restaurants tend to serve large portions, and the food can be high in fat. Plus, there's often a limited choice of vegetables. "Picking the type of restaurant wisely can help," says Hope Warshaw, R.D., author of *Eat Out, Eat Right*. Warshaw says that Asian cuisine—Chinese, Thai, and Vietnamese—generally includes more vegetables.

Hitting Your Stride

The Slugger, Miguel Cabrera, 21

Winning a World Series ring and playing Yankee-killer, all in your rookie season, could make you feel immortal. But Florida Marlin Miguel Cabrera's not buying it. He understands that he has to preserve flexibility while he's young, when he has the tools to do it.

"The secret to my fitness is stretching," says Cabrera. "Before I even hit the weight room, I do my stretching routine, then eight 100-meter sprints." He works a different muscle group every day, paying particular attention to his legs. He climbs stairs and does speed drills that require him to move his feet quickly. And he stretches for 5 minutes after he lifts.

That means Cabrera's muscles are supple enough for him to avoid soothing body treatments. "I try to teach my body to stay healthy on its own," he says. "I don't want to make a habit of ice and massages." That way he can save the ice for more important things—like filling champagne buckets come October.

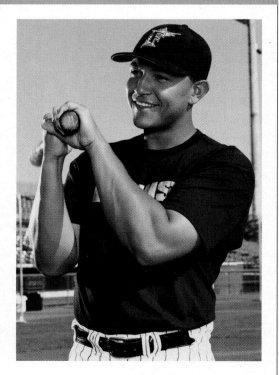

Play hide-and-seek. Put the beer and sodas in your refrigerator's vegetable drawer and leave the carrots out in plain sight so you'll remember to eat them, says Nancy Clark, M.S., R.D., senior sports nutritionist at Boston-based Healthworks Fitness Center.

THE BUFF FACTOR

Looking good can help you land a better job and a better mate. In a recent study, researchers at Yale University found that a significant bias against overweight people—stereotyping them as lazy, less valuable, and less intelligent—exists even among health professionals whose careers emphasize obesity research. So imagine what that Fortune 500 HR specialist thinks.

The Fix

Build your show muscles. Pay particular attention to your chest, shoulders, and biceps—the muscles people are most apt to notice first. To build maximum muscle in these areas, Tom Seabourne, Ph.D., C.S.C.S., an exercise physiologist at Northeastern Texas Community College, designed an exclusive strength-training routine (below) for men in their 20s. It includes explosive power moves, like the bench-press throw, that take advantage of your increased hormonal activity to develop muscle faster.

20s WORKOUT

Perform this workout 2 days a week. Do two or three sets of six to eight repetitions, starting with a weight that's about 30 to 50 percent of your one-rep max for the

---

Time's Toll

The average guy's body fat is . . .

17 percent in his 20s

20 percent in his 30s

22 percent in his 40s

23 percent in his 50s

24 percent in his 60s

That's a 43 percent jump from a man's 20s to his 60s.

---

throws and squats, and 70 to 85 percent for other exercises. Perform the throws and jump squats as fast as you can; for the others, take 2 seconds up, 4 seconds down.

Jump squat

Bench-press throw (on Smith machine)

Straight-bar biceps curl

Stiff-legged deadlift

Shoulder press

Lat pulldown

Hanging knee raise (work up to 20 reps)

Age 30 to 39: Prevention and Planning

Carefree days have been replaced by 24/7 responsibilities: a wife, a baby, a mortgage, and a boss who reminds you of all three. Burritos that disappeared in a puff of metabolic smoke now linger like an oil spill. "Your physiological capacity—the overall performance of most of your body's systems—decreases by around 1 percent per year from

30 onward," says Hayflick. Hence the burrito hangover.

To counter this physiological decline, switch your strategy to preventive fitness. You need to continue lifting heavy weights to preserve the muscle you built in your 20s; stretching takes priority, because you're going to start losing flexibility; and regular interval training is on the list so you can combat the loss of stamina that will start in the middle of this decade. The good news: It's never too late to make a fresh start.

The Changes
NO MORE MR. GUMBY

Flexibility decreases in your 30s, not only because you're likely to sit in an office chair for hours every day, but also because many of the activities you do—running, weight lifting, even basketball—don't call for a full range of motion. "There's actually a shortening of both muscle and connective tissue," says Brent Feland, Ph.D., an aging and flexibility researcher at Brigham Young University.

Life's a Beach

The Sex Star, Jason Lewis, 32

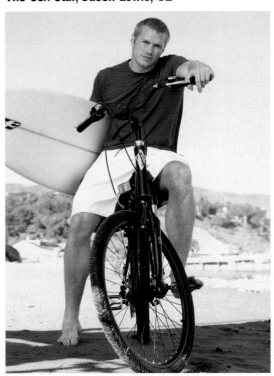

The playground is a distant memory. But that doesn't mean fitness can't be fun. "I play every day, whenever my body and time allow me to," says 32-year-old Jason Lewis, fresh off his starring role in *Sex and the City*. "I love running up gorges and creeks. It's not a predetermined path, so your body has to work in unexpected ways."

He adds an element of surprise in his weight room as well, focusing on exercises with a Swiss ball or medicine ball. Try one of Lewis' favorite ab routines with a workout partner: Grab a medicine ball and sit on the floor. Lift your legs and lean back, so your body forms a V. Now toss the medicine ball with a high loft to your partner, who's in the same position in front of you. Catch the return toss in front of your chest, twist your torso to one side and down, then twist forward as you toss the ball back to your partner. Alternate twisting from side to side.

Of course, this shock-your-body approach to fitness can tear down muscles, so Lewis takes L-glutamine to help his recovery "I'll put it in my water when I go out on my mountain bike," he says.

The Fix

Say yes to yoga. "Yoga requires you to go through full ranges of motion and to hold those positions," says Feland. Take a class once a week and use the moves everywhere. "Get out of your chair and into a stretch while you're watching *SportsCenter*," advises Feland. "It's really easy to do. You just have to develop the habit."

YOUR BEATIN' HEART

Stamina peaks for most men around 31 or 32, but within the next 5 years your aerobic capacity declines. "The heart is a muscle just like any other, and as you age, you lose some strength," says Jordan Metzl, M.D., author of *The Young Athlete: A Sports Doctor's Complete Guide for Parents*. Also starting in your 30s, your body's ability to extract oxygen from your blood diminishes, your cholesterol counts and blood pressure rise, and fatty deposits begin to build up on the walls of your arteries.

The Fix

Schedule a checkup. Ask your doctor to work up your lipoprotein profile. Catch the trouble early enough and it's a good bet that exercise alone will prolong your life.

Speed up, slow down. Maintain your aerobic capacity with regular interval training, says Metzl. Do this workout three times a week: Start with a 10-minute warmup of light jogging. Then sprint for 45 seconds at 80 percent of your maximum heart rate. Recover with 90 seconds of walking or light jogging, and repeat your cycle of sprints

8 to 12 times. Cool down with a 10-minute jog.

PUTTING ON POUNDS

"If your body were a car, it'd require less gas to run as it grew older," says Metzl. In fact, your body consumes 12 fewer calories per day for each year after 30, and most men reach their maximum body weight between ages 34 and 54.

The Fix

Limit your fuel. You need less fuel now, so don't feel obligated to clean your plate at every meal—leave that to the dishwasher. When you snack, don't eat from the box or carton. If you dole out a reasonable portion, you'll be less likely to absentmindedly eat the whole container.

MISSING MUSCLE

Electrical forces bind all of your body's molecules together, but these forces begin to weaken in your 30s, so some of those molecules begin to malfunction. Strength and coordination are usually the first to go, and muscle mass drops. If you don't take steps to prevent it, you'll lose about 6 pounds of muscle in the next 10 years.

The Fix

Build muscle for daily activities. Switch focus from mirror muscles to functional strength, flexibility, and balance. Your tendons and joints aren't as sturdy as they used to be when you were a kid; pay attention to form to prevent injuries. Seabourne's slow-tempo exercises (see page 206) are safer for your joints, but you'll still maintain a high intensity.

30s WORKOUT

Perform this workout 2 or 3 days a week. Do 2 or 3 sets of 8 to 10 repetitions, starting with 75 percent of your one-rep maximum. If you can do more than 12 reps, you're not lifting enough weight. If your form worsens before 10 reps, use a lighter weight. The tempo for all of these is 2 seconds up, 4 seconds down.

Dumbell lunge: You'll put less strain on your knees if you take large steps and make sure your front knee is lined up directly over (not past) your toes.

Cable fly: Bend forward slightly from the hips, and keep your shoulders pressed down and back.

Seated leg curl: Don't allow your back to lift off the pad.

Bent-over row: Tighten your abs, bend at the hips, and keep your back flat.

Time's Toll

The average guy can sit and reach . . .

17.5 inches (2.5 inches beyond his toes) in his 20s

16.5 inches (1.5 inches beyond his toes) in his 30s

15.3 inches (0.3 inches beyond his toes) in his 40s

14.5 inches (within 0.5 inches of his toes) in his 50s

13.5 inches (within 1.5 inches of his toes) in his 60s

The average man's flexibility (as measured by reach length) shrinks by 23 percent from his 20s to his 60s.

Reverse curl: Don't bring your forearm beyond perpendicular to the floor.

Situp on situp board: Hook your feet under the ankle pads. Bend your knees slightly, and do a full situp through the entire range of motion. Or do Swiss-ball crunches.

Age 40 to 49: Never Back Down

During your 40s, you realize that your body's warranty has indeed expired. And you could probably use a little body work. "All my buddies are getting fat," says 48-year-old Seabourne, the author of *Athletic Abs: Maximum Core Fitness Training*. But your 40s are also when you've established your career a bit, so you can leave the late-night duty to junior staff. For the first time since college, you have a little discretionary time. You've earned 3 hours of workout time during the week and a longer session on the weekends. No excuses. Your body needs the work right now; delay isn't an option.

The Changes
THE INCREDIBLE SHRINKING YOU

For most men in their 40s, height begins to decrease. "Disks in the spine are fluid filled, like shock absorbers," says Seabourne. "But as you grow older, they act more like dried-out sponges." By the time you hit 60, you'll likely have shrunk by $1^1/_4$ inches.

The Fix

Stand and sit up straight. Seabourne says posture is more important now than ever. Imagine you have a string pulling your body up from the top of your head: shoulders back, head up, spine neutral. "That'll keep those disks healthy. And you'll appear thinner and taller because your posture will be better," he says.

Lengthen and strengthen. Developing the muscular endurance of your core is essential to maintaining good posture, says Seabourne. The key is to lengthen your spine through stretching, and strengthening your abs and lower back. Try to do this exercise at least once every day:

The yoga pose. Stand with your feet shoulder-width apart, and place your hands against the small of your back. Inhale as you slowly lift your chest. Exhale as you stretch, slowly tilting your head back and gently pulling your elbows toward each other. Remain in this position, and let gravity stretch you into the natural arch of your back. Do this for 3 to 8 seconds. Try it between sets of your weight workout.

SORE SUBJECT

Whatever your sport, you have to prepare your body to perform. Lots of middle-aged weekend warriors come home with injuries like torn hamstrings, sprained ankles, or worse.

The Fix

Feel the flow. Seabourne says a short warmup—8 to 10 minutes of light cardiovascular work—starts the flow of synovial fluid, a natural lubricating solution found in joints. It also elevates your core temperature so your muscles are more elastic and you have less chance of injury.

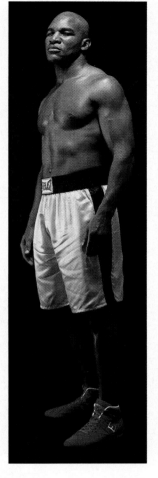

Punch the Clock

The Champ, Evander Holyfield, 41

"As far as working out, I know exactly what I'm doing," says Evander Holyfield. No argument here: Just look at the man and those three heavyweight championship belts.

But even he has challenges. "At the times I need to be reacting, I'm thinking more," he says. "When I was younger, I didn't have to concentrate as much. It was just fun."

Holyfield prepares better now, so when it's time to act, he's confident in his abilities. "I spend more time warming up, more time stretching. And I pray a lot," he says. "That's how I prepare myself mentally."

He prepares himself nutritionally by eating well before workouts. "Sugar leaves you stranded; I make sure I have the proper amount of protein before I work out."

Of course, prep work will get you nowhere if you do it only occasionally. Holyfield trains 3 days a week; he ups it to 5 days when he's training for a fight. "Consistency is key. I believe it's easier to maintain than to rebuild."

AGE-OLD PROBLEMS

As your personal odometer ticks upward, your risks of heart attack, stroke, and high blood pressure also go up. You owe it to yourself and your family to stick to an exercise program—the best way to dodge heart and head bombs. But to keep in the game, you have to prepare your body to perform. The day after exercise, you want to feel a pleasant soreness, not debilitating injuries.

The Fix

Find a trail. A study of nearly 11,000 Harvard alumni found that a brisk 30- to 60-minute walk 5 days a week cuts stroke risk by 24 to 50 percent.

Keep track. Get credit for every step you take with the Garmin Foretrex 201 ($180), which keeps track of your speed, distance, and pace. Don't worry about getting lost; the built-in GPS will guide you back home again. (In your 40s, your memory declines as well.)

A Chip Shot to 50

The Shark, Greg Norman, 49

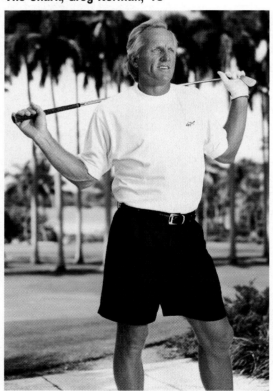

Know this about predators: They're easily triggered into attack mode. "I'm appalled by people who don't look after their bodies," snarls Greg Norman. You can't go slack just because your birthday candles now set off the home fire alarm. The 49-year-old golf champ points out that as you make the turn to life's back nine, abs are an absolute necessity. "I've had problems with my back because in my 20s and early 30s I never worked on my abs or my back," he says.

He's now on the road 40 weeks a year, so he had no more time than you do to bust a gut. His solution: He travels and trains with a Swiss ball and tubing to strengthen his core and rotator cuffs, and to maintain flexibility.

He's been a muscle-building enthusiast since long before it was popular for golfers. "When I was a kid, we were told that exercising was bad for your golf swing," he says. "I was the one who first changed all that." Now 85 percent of tour players follow regular strength-training programs, according to Norman. "My family's the same way, so it's easy for all of us to self-regulate. I'm aware of my body because I want to be around a long time."

LESS MUSCLE = MORE FAT

"After age 30, you lose about half a pound of muscle per year—if you're sedentary—which turns into 2.6 pounds of fat per year, just because of metabolic slowdown," says Seabourne. In that trade-off, everybody loses.

The Fix

Eat six small meals daily instead of three big ones. It'll keep your furnace stoked, making it burn fat more efficiently. It'll also boost HDL (good) cholesterol and cut LDL (bad) cholesterol.

Add a pound of muscle. Muscle tissue needs more calories for maintenance and re-building processes than fat tissue does. The more muscle you have, the more calories you burn—even at rest. "Gain just 1 pound of muscle, and that's an additional 50 calories you'll burn each day," says Seabourne. For the 40s strength workout (below), Seabourne calls for a slower lifting tempo but keeps the weights fairly heavy, so you can build muscle mass. "It's still cool to lift heavy, but you need to pay strict attention to your form and protect your joints," he says. Glucosamine supplements can help with your day-after pains.

40s WORKOUT

Perform this workout 2 days a week. Do 2 or 3 sets of 10 to 12 reps, starting with 70 percent of your one-rep max. If you can do more than 12 reps, you're not lifting enough weight. If you lose your form before 12 reps, use a lighter weight. Take 2 seconds going up, 6 seconds down.

Barbell squat

Dumbbell bench press

Dumbbell shoulder press (or Arnold press)

Seated row

Incline biceps curl

Standing calf raise

Russian twist (start with 15 reps to each side; build up to 25)

Age 49 and Up: Defending Your Turf

By now you have it figured out (i.e., you know that nobody has it figured out). You're a master at the office, a veteran in the weight room, the head of the clan. But you're fighting Mother Nature and entropy at the same time, and that's one tough tag team. Australian researchers found that men age 58 and older often struggle with body-image issues. Performing at least two exercise sessions per week boosts men's self-esteem by helping them feel better about their bodies' ability to perform routine tasks. And feeling good motivates you to make more gains. Your fitness program should help you avoid pain and do what's important to you. Okay, so you're not a kid anymore. Neither is Clint Eastwood. But he can still kick some butt.

The Changes
THAT TRICK KNEE JUST GOT TRICKIER

Many men in their 50s begin to have joint trouble. The main culprits: overuse injuries and osteoarthritis.

Time's Toll

The average guy jumps . . .

20.5 inches high in his 20s

19.5 inches high in his 30s

16 inches high in his 40s

14 inches high in his 50s

The average man's explosive power declines by 32 percent from his 20s to his 50s.

The Fix

Ride a bike. Researchers at Arcadia University in Glenside, Pennsylvania, studied 39 people suffering from osteoarthritis of the knees and found that cycling just 25 minutes a day, three times a week, significantly improved pain relief and performance in walking tests. So saddle up.

BONE LOSS LOOMS

Bone minerals are lost and replaced throughout life—it's a natural process—but after age 35, the loss begins to outpace the replacement. By age 50, this imbalance can hurt you.

The Fix

More stress. Stressing your bones strengthens them. Walking beats swimming, running beats walking, and strength training is the best bone builder of all, says Wojtek Chodzko-Zajko, Ph.D., head of kinesiology at the University of Illinois.

Have a cow. The average 50-year-old needs about 1,200 milligrams (mg) of calcium per day for healthy bones. Get that from one 8-ounce glass of milk (300 mg),

6 ounces of yogurt (300 mg), a handful of almonds (150 mg), and 2 ounces of Swiss cheese (540 mg).

OH, MY ACHING BACK

Inactivity can tighten your spine and pelvic muscles, forcing your knees and lower back to compensate. That's why they ache, explains Mark Verstegen, author of *Core Performance.*

The Fix

Roll your foam. Exercising with a foam roll can loosen the muscles around your pelvis and torso. You can purchase one at therapyzone.com. Lie on top of the roll with your arms crossed over your chest. Keep your abs tight and your feet on the ground. Glide on the roll from your shoulders to the base of your spine several times until you feel the muscles release.

Take a Pilates class. Strengthening your stomach muscles can ease back pain. "Pilates includes a lot of balance activities on one hand and one knee that are aimed at stabilizing and strengthening the core," says Chodzko-Zajko. Call (800) 474-5283 to find a Pilates studio near you.

WATER SHORTAGE

Between ages 57 and 86, your body literally dries up. It will likely consist of just 54 percent water, as opposed to the 61 percent found in younger men. You'll also sweat less because your sweat glands disappear. You may have less body odor, but overheating and heatstroke become an issue.

The Fix

Be a camel. "Drinking fluids is more important as you grow older," says Chodzko-Zajko. "One of the problems with aging is that thirst decreases with age, so people tend to drink less."

MASS DEFECTIONS

You've been trying to lose flab for 2 decades, but now your body is doing it on its own. Unfortunately, between 50 and 80 you may also lose 35 percent of your muscle mass.

The Fix

Play with heavy metal. Don't shy away from heavy weights because you think you're susceptible to injury. As long as you use proper form, which you should master now if you haven't already, heavy weights will keep your bones strong and your muscles large. Seabourne kept the weights up in your workout (below) but slowed the tempo and concentrated on lifts that develop balance. This way, you won't be knocked off-kilter when the bank hands over your 401(k) payout.

50s WORKOUT

Perform this workout 2 days a week. Do 2 or 3 sets of 10 to 15 repetitions, starting with 65 percent of your one-rep max. If you can do more than 15 reps, you're not lifting enough weight. If you lose your form before 10 reps, use a lighter weight. Keep the speed at 6 seconds up, 6 seconds down.

One-legged half squat (begin without weight)

One-legged deadlift (with or without weight)

One-arm row (on low cable pulley)

Lateral raise and front raise

Standing alternating arm curl

Lying dumbbell pullover

Standing overhead medicine-ball throw (against a wall or with a partner)

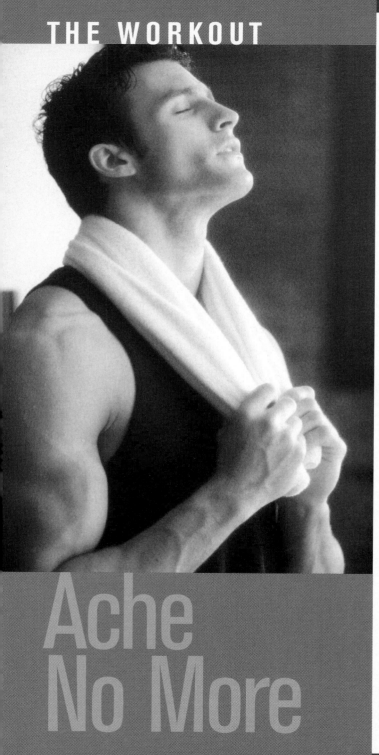

Ache No More

The older you get, the more your body hurts. Here's a proven program for beating wear and tear and staying in great shape

I'm 45 years old, and I played football throughout high school and college. Now I run. Not fast, not far, but I run. And my joints have paid the price. Over the past 25 years, I've probably tried 40 workout routines, with varying degrees of success. The following program is the only one I have time for nowadays (due to job and family time and a yard full of weeds that seem to be on steroids), but it's enough. My workout makes me feel better. I don't hurt much, and I have more energy. I bet it'll work for you, too.

Loosen Up

If I try to stretch and do my abs-and-back routine at the gym, I find I don't have time for much lifting. So I do that stuff at home while I watch the evening news. It gives me a feeling of accomplishment and control while watching news I can be only a passive (and somber) consumer of. It's a ritual: hamstrings, back, groin, shoulders, 50 crunches, 50 twisting crunches, then bird dogs (see photo). This one you may not know. It works the muscles directly opposite your abs: the lower- and middle-back extensors. I love this exercise because it builds flexibility and back strength—and it always brings a smile to my wife's face. "Good boy. Roll over, Rover," she teases.

BY JEFF CSATARI

Lose Weight

On weekdays when I don't lift (Tuesdays and Fridays), I do 20 to 45 minutes of aerobic activity (depending on how much time I have). I jump on whatever's free at the gym: stationary bike, elliptical trainer, or treadmill. If they're all tied up, I jump rope. On Wednesdays I try to play basketball with the guys at work. On weekends, I tackle yard work and home repairs. If it's raining, I'll carry 40-pound bags of water-softener salt up and down the stairs 10 times. My wife sees no logic in this, but it gets my heart rate up quick.

Build Strength

Thirty minutes of weight training two times a week is all I really need. I'm long past trying to impress bachelorettes with my muscles. I just want a body that works and doesn't hurt. I hit chest, shoulders, and triceps one day, and legs and back the next time I lift. I do the basics: bench presses, triceps kickbacks, lightweight flies (for my creaky shoulders), dumbbell twisting standing shoulder presses (see photos), calf raises, and leg presses or squats. Two of my favorite lifts are the barbell front squat and the Romanian deadlift with bent-over row (again, see photos) because they target my most useful muscles—in my legs and back. One more thing: I've found that the older I get, the more I need to warm up, 10 minutes at least. But you can let breaking a sweat be your guide.

BIRD DOG

● Start on all fours, with your knees and toes on the floor and your palms facedown in front of you. Pull in your abs; then straighten one arm and the opposite leg, extending both limbs until they're parallel to the floor. Keep your torso and hips in a straight line. Hold for 5 seconds, then return to the starting position and repeat with the opposite arm and leg.

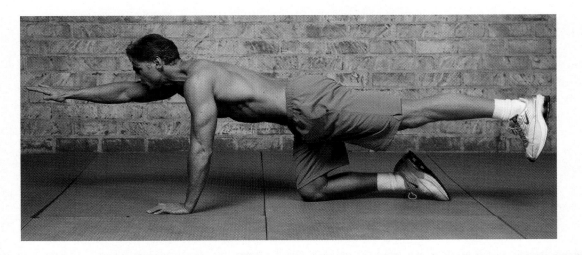

TWISTING STANDING SHOULDER PRESS

● Stand while holding a pair of dumbbells just outside your shoulders at jaw level, palms facing in.

● Press the dumbbells overhead as you turn to your right. Lower the dumbbells as you turn back to the center. Press them up again as you turn to the left, then lower them as you return to the starting position.

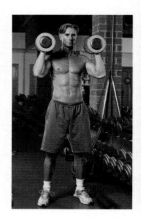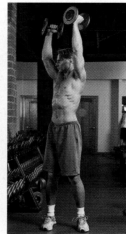

BARBELL FRONT SQUAT

● Grab the barbell with an overhand grip, hands just beyond shoulder width, and hold it in front of you, just above your shoulders. Raise your upper arms so they're parallel to the floor while letting the bar roll back onto your fingers (not your palms). Your feet should be shoulder-width apart, knees slightly bent. Keep your back straight and your eyes focused straight ahead.

● Without changing the position of your arms, lower your body until your thighs are parallel to the floor. Pause, then push yourself back up to the starting position.

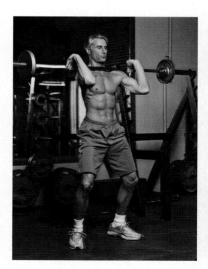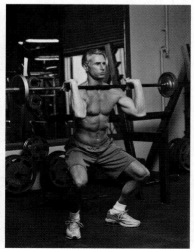

ROMANIAN DEADLIFT WITH BENT-OVER ROW

● Grab the barbell with a shoulder-width over-hand grip, and hold it at arm's length in front of your thighs. Your feet should be shoulder-width apart, your knees slightly bent, and your shoulders pulled back.

● Bend over at the hips to lower the bar down your legs, toward the floor. Stop when your torso is parallel to the floor or when you can't go lower without rounding your back. Pause.

● From this position, do a bent-over row. Without moving your torso, squeeze your shoulder blades together and pull the bar to your chest. Pause, then lower it. Stand to return to the starting position.

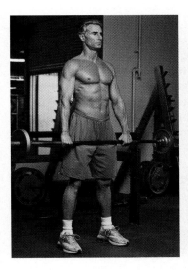
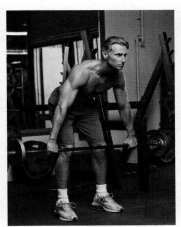
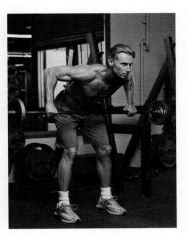

TRAINING TIPS

Q I've been diagnosed with shoulder impingement. My doctor said to avoid exercises that hurt the shoulder. Do I have to quit lifting?

M.A., DAYTON, OHIO

A No. The smartest trainers we know uniformly hammer home the need for middle-back strength. The key is to emphasize what these trainers consider the most important movement: scapular retraction, or pulling your shoulder blades together.

Try this: In a horizontal-row or seated-chest-press machine, put the seat higher than normal, so the bar or grips are lower than normal. Pull your shoulder blades together, taking care not to shrug them upward. Now a row or press should be pain-free.

TOUGH TALK

"Any workout which does not involve a certain minimum of danger or responsibility does not improve the body—it just wears it out."

NORMAN MAILER

Q I rolled my ankle pretty badly during a paintball game. The doc at the walk-in clinic said I didn't need to support it, but my regular doctor put me in an air cast. Which is better, immobilizing or not?

C.W., GARY, INDIANA

A This sounds like a classic sprain, in which the ligaments on the outside of the joint get stretched or torn. There are three classifications of sprains: mild, moderate, and severe. Typically you don't need to immobilize the ankle unless the injury is severe and you've torn all of the ligaments. Air casts are sometimes used to support the ankle early in the healing phase, but aren't always necessary. For mild and moderate sprains, it's im-

TEE OFF

Put Off Hip Replacement

If you like to swing iron when you're not lifting it, you may be at risk of tearing cartilage in your hip. In a recent University of Pittsburgh study, researchers took MRIs of eight golfers with hip pain and found that each had a torn labrum, the cartilage that stabilizes the hip joint. "Golfers focus on rotator-cuff and trunk-rotation exercises, but it's the hips that are most often injured," says Scott Lephart, Ph.D., one of the study authors. To help prevent a tear, balance on one leg for 20 seconds with your eyes open and then again with your eyes closed. Do this three times on each leg before you tee off.

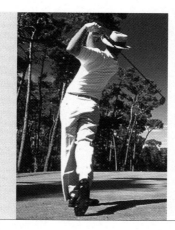

Sidestep Ankle Sprains

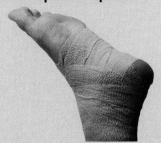

Having textured insole in your shoes may reduce your risk of ankle injury when you run or play sports. Researchers in Australia performed a series of experiments on 17 soccer players, testing their foot sensitivity and balance. In some trials, the players were barefoot, and in others they wore either regular soccer cleats or shoes with textured insoles. "Smooth soles appear to impair balance, making it harder to tell what kind of footing you've got and increasing risk of ankle injury," says Gordon Waddington, Ph.D., the study author. In contrast, nubby insoles improve sensation and balance almost to the level you experience when going barefoot, he says.

portant to resume light activity to maintain your range of motion—so immobilization isn't advisable. But don't rush off to the paintball field. Anti-inflammatory medications will help with the swelling, but these injuries need time to heal. By the way, did you win?

Q After a 2-hour workout (much longer than usual), I felt shaky. The next day I woke up feeling hungover and too nauseated to eat. What's going on?

J.B., ORONO, MAINE

Use Your Noggin

Percentage by which wearing a bike helmet reduces your risk of serious head and brain injury:

85

A You're shaky, dizzy, and nauseated because your body is telling you to chill out—you're dehydrated and have too much lactic acid in your system. You should be well hydrated before strenuous workouts and have a little food in your stomach (try a

Help Your Hinges

Knees hurt? Bad elbow? Lifting weights may ease the pain of sore, stiff joints. Tufts University researchers had men and women with knee pain perform weight-bearing exercises, such as squats and leg extensions, regularly for 4 months. At the end of the trial, the lifters were able to stand, walk, and climb stairs more easily and had up to 43 percent less joint pain than when the trial began. "Muscles

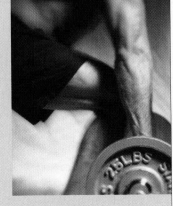

act as shock absorbers for joints, so the more in shape your muscles are, the more they protect your joints and keep them from hurting," says Ronenn Roubenoff, M.D., one of the study authors.

piece of fruit). Working out too hard for too long can deplete your electrolyte stores and lead to cramping and nausea. If you insist on doing a long workout, prep with fluids and food.

BACK ON THE FAIRWAY

I hurt my back last year. Now I want to play golf again. Can I do it safely?
A.C., CHARLOTTE, NORTH CAROLINA

It's important to loosen up your back before a round of golf. While standing, bend at the waist and dangle your arms. Hold for 30 seconds, then slowly straighten up. Do this five times. Next, swing your driver 20 times like a baseball bat while rotating

your hips, starting with your elbows in, then gradually extending your arms.

BATTLE OF THE BULGE

After I did situps recently, the area around my left testicle felt bruised. Maybe a groin pull?
G.T., IRVINE, CALIFORNIA

That, or it's possible you've developed a hernia from repetitive straining due to bad situp form—like keeping one side contracted for too long. The stress on your abdominal muscles can cause the intestines to bulge through a weakness in the groin. My advice is to visit your doctor—only he can put his

finger in just the right spot to detect this. Your condition doesn't sound like a groin pull, as you'd be feeling soreness when you stretch the area while walking or exercising—not after situps.

OFF THE CUFF

Best Move for Rotator Cuff
Researchers at the Steadman-Hawkins Sports Medicine Foundation in Colorado measured the muscle activity in 15 participants performing different exercises aimed at rehabilitating the upper subscapularis—the rotator-cuff muscle involved in throwing. The winner? This exercise: Grab a light dumbbell

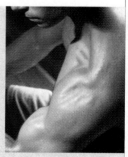

and, with your elbow a few inches from your side, bend your arm so it forms a 90-degree angle. Slowly rotate your forearm until the dumbbell touches your chest, pause, then rotate back.

PAIN RELIEVER

For a pulled muscle, can I take Advil in one big dose and really knock back the pain?
P.R., HOUMA, LOUISIANA

There's a reason the bottle comes with directions. Taking one big dose won't help, but it can hurt—with side effects like diarrhea, nausea, and stomach ulcers. Follow the dosing directions, and spread it over the day. The directions may seem conservative, but that's so people don't do damage by taking too much. If the standard 200 milligrams doesn't do much for you, call your M.D. to see if it's safe to take a higher dose. And while ibuprofen may relieve the pain, it won't do anything to heal any muscle damage. To speed the repair, take 1,000 international units of vitamin E until you feel like your old self again.

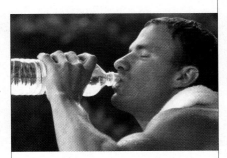

Muscle Mishaps

Apparently, we're practically killing ourselves to get ripped. In a recent University of Arkansas study, researchers identified 20,489 weight-training injuries over a 20-year period and determined that two in every three stemmed from the improper use of equipment. The most-often injured part of the body? The hands. Protect your mitts—and the rest of you—with these fixes for the most common weight-room flubs, courtesy of Dave Tate, C.S.C.S, owner of Elite Fitness Systems in London, Ohio.

INJURED AREA	PERCENTAGE OF ALL INJURIES	HOW TO PREVENT . . .
Hands (includes wrists)	23.8	**Hyperextension-Induced Strains:** Keep the barbell in line with your forearms during bench presses and arm curls; don't bend your hands back.
Upper Trunk (includes shoulders)	18.8	**Muscle Pulls, Irritated Rotator Cuffs:** Keep your elbows in, not flared out, on the bench press to prevent overrotation of the shoulder joint.
Head (includes neck and upper trapezius)	16.4	**Neck Strains:** Keep your head neutral rather than pushing it into the pad on machines.
Lower Trunk (includes abs)	15.5	**Lower-Back Strains:** Keep your abs in and your back flat when doing bent-over rows.
Feet	14.6	**Broken or Fractured Bones:** Pay attention when removing a large plate from a barbell; you could miss the smaller plates in front of it and drop one on your foot.
Arms	5.3	**Muscle Pulls:** Use moderate weights until you develop enough muscle mass to go heavier.
Legs	4.9	**Knee Sprains:** Don't let your knee go in front of your toes when doing lunges or using a leg-press machine.

Credits

Cover Photo Credit
© Wes Bell

Interior Photo Credits
© Ondrea Barbe: page 128
© John Biever/Sports Illustrated: page 190
© Beth Bischoff: pages iv (back), 21, 26, 27, 28, 29, 30, 31, 32, 33, 34, 35, 36, 37, 38, 39, 49, 52, 53, 54, 58, 59, 65, 66, 67, 68, 69, 72, 73, 74, 75, 76, 77, 78, 79, 93, 94, 95, 96, 97, 98, 99, 102, 104, 105, 106, 107 (exercise series), 109, 110, 111, 113, 114, 115, 118, 119, 120, 121, 122, 123, 124, 125, 127 (exercise series), 141, 142, 143, 144, 151, 152, 153, 154, 155, 156, 157, 158, 159, 160, 161, 162, 163, 164, 188, 189, 198, 199
© Brand X Pictures: page 126
© E. J. Camp: page 204
© Ron Chapple/Taxi/Getty Images: page 80
© Photographer's Choice: page 172
© Rich Clarkson/Allsport/Getty Images: page 184 (Louganis)
© Bettman Corbis: page 184 (bullfighter)
© Joseph Cultice: pages 200, 208
© EMPICS/Sportschrome: page 145
© Darryl Estrine: pages iii (back), iv (lunge, weight lifting), 41, 46, 48, 55, 101, 108, 207
© Annie Etheridge: page 62 (left, right)
© Nicholas Eveleigh: page 176
© Macduff Everton/Corbis: page 216
© Eyewire: page 40 (wristwatch)
© Jon Feingersh/Corbis: pages iii (running), 139
© Andrew French: pages 174, 175
John Hamel/Rodale Images: pages 81, 83, 134
© Mark Hanauer: pages 213, 214, 215
© Mark Havriliak: pages 60, 70, 86, 90, 195
Hilmar: page 166
Rodale Images: page 40 (cereal)
© Monte Isom: page 92
© Dave Krieger: pages 130, 132, 135, 194
© Nick Laham/Getty Images: page 192

© Robert Lewis: pages 15, 19
© Svend Lindbaek: page 100
© Steven Lippman: pages x, 11, 25, 44, 70, 84, 116, 150
Mitch Mandel/Rodale Images: pages 6, 13, 22, 23, 24, 43 (Burger King, Taco Bell), 62 (center), 82, 217 (exercise), 218
© John Manno: pages 5, 10, 43 (Boston Market)
© Craig Melvin: page 184 (Malarchuk)
© Sean Murphy: pages 146, 148
© Erin Patrice O'Brien: page 202
© Jose Luis Pelaez/Corbis: page 212
© PhotoDisc: page 217 (foot)
© Tom Rafalovich: page 170
© Chip Simons/Taxi/Getty Images: page 2
Margaret Skrovanek/Rodale Images: page 219
© Chuck Solomon/Sports Illustrated: pages 185 (Florie), 193
© Bob Straus: page 184 (Janovich)
© Stockbyte: pages 127 (close up), 171
© Thinkstock: page 112
© AP Wide World Photos: pages iv (players colliding), 180, 181, 184 (Tittle, Kendall), 185 (Saunders, Theisman), 187
Kurt Wilson/Rodale Images: page 168
© John G. Zimmerman/Sports Illustrated: page 185 (Gifford)

Ebonite bowling ball (bottom) courtesy of Bowlersparadise.com: page 9
Storm Hit bowling ball (top) courtesy of Bowling.com: page 9
Courtesy of Bridgestone: page 7

Interior Illustration Credits
© Molly Borman/Darryl Estrine: page 107 (chest muscles)
© Mark Matcho: page 165
© Quade Paul: page 196

Index